AGING WISELY
AND LIVING LONGER:
A PERSONAL JOURNEY

Yosh Taguchi

B.Sc. Psychology, McGill, 1955
MDCM, McGill, 1959
FRCS(C) 1964
PhD, Investigative Medicine, McGill, 1970

D1453828

This book was published with the assistance of
CanamBooks self-publishing services.

Printed in Canada

Paperback: 978-1-7773575-0-4
Ebook (EPUB): 978-1-7773575-1-1
Ebook (MOBI): 978-1-7773575-2-8

Editor: Lisa Audrey Cohen

Design: Ted Sancton/Studio Melrose

This book was set in Scala Pro 12/16

"My mind then wandered. I thought of this: I thought of how ever day each of us experiences a few little moments that have just a bit more resonance than other moments. We hear a word that sticks in our mind or maybe have a small experience that pulls us out of ourselves, if only briefly... and if we were to collect these small moments in a notebook and save them over a period of months, we would see certain trends emerge from our collection; certain voices would emerge that have been trying to speak through us.

We would realize that we have been having another life altogether, one we didn't even know was going on inside us. And maybe this other life is more important than the one we think of as being real; this clunky day to day world of furniture and noise and metal. So just maybe it is these small silent moments which are the true story-making events of our lives."

DOUGLAS COUPLAND, *Life After God*

This book is dedicated to
VALERIA ROSENBLOOM,
for her support and friendship
in good times and bad,
and in memory of her late husband,
my dear friend,
MIKE ROSENBLOOM

Contents

Prologue

My name is Yosh Taguchi and as a urologic surgeon, I have been involved in thousands of lives in a career that spans over five decades.

I have sat in my office across from patients and their loved ones and I have had to say the three words no one wants to hear: "You have cancer." I have also had the privilege of being able to say: "You are cured."

I have looked into each of their eyes and have seen the sadness, the fear, the wonderment of how this could possibly be happening to them.

I was able to tell the family (as they paced up and down for hours upon hours); that their loved one survived the surgery and that I was pleased with how the surgery went.

I have come out of surgery and have had to inform the family (and later the patient), that when I opened them up, there was so much damage already done. I would not be able to alter the course of the illness. It would be fatal. "How much time?", they would inevitably ask, all I could do was provide a realm of possibilities.

With my gift and ability as a surgeon, I have sculpted diseased parts to a new and improved form. In doing so, I have held both life and death in my hands.

I faced possible death myself, having had cardiac bypass surgery more than ten years ago. I became the patient and my family became the people pacing up and down wondering "What if?"

Now, in my 8th decade, I find my heart dancing upon my soul, to the beat of life's intricate balance between the beginning, the middle and the end.

Introduction

I can say that my worst experiences in the operating room have been times removing kidneys from brain dead donors whose heart is still very much alive and the body protesting, and in cancer surgery when blood loss is severe and seemingly out of control. The exhilarating moments are when difficult cancer surgery proceeds better than even imagined.

I remember assisting a resident trying to remove a cancerous right kidney. The bleeding was getting out of control and he signalled with his eyes that he would like me take over. I dissected the area between the vena cava (the main vein) and the aorta (the main artery) at the level of the kidney and clamped the right renal artery going under the big main vein. That stopped the bleeding and allowed the resident to complete the surgery.

"Very nicely done!" said the resident.

"Remember that when you are in trouble with the right kidney," I replied.

The most memorable case I ever had in my career occurred in my first year in practice. A woman in her late thirties was admitted to my care from the emergency room because I was the urologist on call. She had tried to terminate a pregnancy because she already had three children and her husband had been recently diagnosed with schizophrenia. She had been instructed by friends to terminate the pregnancy by instilling a combination of lye and hydrogen peroxide into her cervix. She managed to instill the caustic fluid into her bladder.

When the doctors in Emergency saw her she was in agony and there was a grey material protruding from her urinary meatus. The doctor clamped the protruding mass, and when he pulled, out came the entire lining of her bladder. Our residents were called and she was admitted under my care.

The logical thing to do was to create a urinary diversion as we do when the entire bladder has to be removed because of an invasive cancer. In the procedure a six inch segment of small intestine is disconnected from the bowel tract. The distal end of the isolated segment is opened to the skin like someone with an ileostomy. The proximal end of the six inch segment is closed and anchored to the back wall of the abdomen. The two tubes from the kidneys, called the ureters are connected to the isolated segment of small intestine. The procedure is known as ileal loop urinary diversion.

We had an open discussion of her case. Why not build her a new bladder using the large intestine in a procedure known as colocystoplasty, I argued. We determined that her urethra, the tube from the bladder to the meatus, was healthy. Our patient agreed to our attempt to try to build her a new bladder. She was made aware that in addition to regular urination she would probably require self-catheterization on a regular basis. She consented. She did very well with the surgery and I followed her regularly for five decades. She became a good friend greeting me on every visit with a warm hug, and her oldest daughter became a wife of a doctor in Europe. Many patients have become lifelong friends.

The most satisfying procedure I have carried out numerous times in my lifetime is the surgical removal of a cancerous prostate with the diagnosis made early enough to assure a lifetime cure. The challenge is to effect a cure while maintaining urine control and a functional erection. I have been the surgeon for several dozen doctors, including three senior surgeons of my hospital in Montreal. Thus it was a shock to be summoned to a meeting by my administrative chief. At the meeting, attended as well by the head of urological oncology, I was asked to stop doing the prostate surgery.

"Why?" I asked.

"You were not specifically trained for the procedure," said the administrative head.

I was stunned and rendered speechless. But the head of urological oncology spoke up:

"But, this is the man who taught us how to do it!" he said.

That ended the meeting! To this day I am puzzled why this encounter ever took place. The fact is: it did! Surgeons do not learn procedures which they simply repeat over and over in their lifetime. Innovations, modifications, and changes for the better have always been part of our daily life.

CHAPTER ONE

To Begin With

I s there a way to age wisely and live longer? We all know people who appear to have discovered the secret. They are well into their eighties, nineties, or even past the century mark and they are alert, walking briskly, going on cruises, enjoying their grandchildren or great grandchildren, and requiring a minimum of medications or, perhaps, none at all! Our first impulse is to assume that they have been blessed with a fortunate genetic endowment and indeed, upon inquiry, many of them appear to have blood relatives who have had very long lives.

But, it's not all in the genes as many experts and scientific studies have now ascertained. Identical twins die, on average, fifteen years apart. Wow! Isn't that startling? Who would have guessed that? I would have thought that identical twins would die months or perhaps, at most, a few years apart. But, fifteen years! That information alone should give us pause and make us wonder about factors other than heredity that affect life-spans. Scientists in the field say genes contribute fifteen to twenty percent to longevity. What, then, makes up the remaining eighty percent?

I am now into the eighth decade of my life: I am eighty-seven years old to be exact. Thus, I have a selfish and personal reason to want to explore this question? It is surprisingly easy to-day to get an answer to a medical question. Google "longevity" or "life span" and there is a mountain of information out there at our fingertips. Anyone with a digital device and access to the internet has an up-to-date encyclopedia at his immediate disposal.

I vowed to make a personal odyssey on this question. What can or should I do to add years to my life? More importantly, how can I add time that is meaningful, invigorating, and worthwhile? How much of the information out there is solid science and how much of it interesting, titillating, even entertaining, perhaps, but actually useless nonsense? How much of it is unscrupulous money grab targeting gullible seniors? Then, it occurred to me that I might be able to take interested parties along with me on this voyage of discovery. There is, after all, nothing like trying to explain something to another person to make it clearer in your own mind.

Although I am a surgeon by training, a retired urologic surgeon, to be exact, I consider myself primarily a teacher. I have been involved in the teaching or training of two or three generations of doctors: how to become better, competent, reliable surgeons of the genitourinary tracts of men and women – a urologist, in short. In the process I have become a better student and a better human being.

The best definition of learning I have come across is this one: "Learning is a process of discovery and remembering what you have discovered." What that says is that every student has to make the discovery for himself: another person, not even the most accomplished, gifted and dedicated teacher cannot do that for him or her. The best a teacher can do is to provide the environment, encourage the effort, and rejoice when the discovery or learning takes place.

Let me set the record straight. I have no intention of overwhelming the reader with academic minutia. In fact, I will only mention information I find interesting and meaningful and I will do so in a conversational tone. For encyclopedic details on the subject go elsewhere. I am going to talk about what I plan to do to live as full and as long a life as I can. I think I am intellectually prepared to do this, but can I actually change my lifestyle at this time in my life? Can I change my eating habits? Can I exercise more? Can I learn to meditate? What else might I be expected to do? This might be fun, but it could be difficult, a self-inflicted torture, in fact. Might I discover, as well, that I have missed the boat, that it is too late for me to make the changes. And then, maybe not.

First, we will examine the various theories of aging. Not all of them, only those I find interesting and in a language we can all understand.

Then, in part two of this endeavor I will examine the most common causes of death in this country and how we might reduce our own risks regarding these disorders, one by one. After all, what's the point of trying to add years of life and have your own life shortened by a killing disorder not appropriately addressed. I should mention here that all the books on aging I have come across largely ignore this question, and I don't know why.

And, finally, in part three, I will take a critical look at the health care industry in Canada of which I have been an intimate part for over half a century. What do I think is good about it and what do I think is not so good about it, and how might we change what we can for the better. Does being a part of the industry allow me to see or suggest changes that can and should be made, or does it blind me from actually observing what might be wrong? What I hope to do as well is to help the reader navigate the complicated system better.

Certainly, at my age and point in life, I cannot be hurt or punished for whatever I may want to say. I have become too old for that. I realize that statements about health care systems and disorderly body functions are not necessarily fascinating subjects for the average reader.

Let's get started!

Are we, in fact, living longer?

It is widely reported that the average lifespan in the developed countries of the world has increased by a decade or two in the past few hundred years so that it is now into the mid-eighties in most developed countries today. But, is average lifespan the parameter we should be looking at? Average lifespan means that every death is counted including infant and maternal deaths at childbirths, childhood deaths from failure of appropriate immunization, youths lost in battle, deaths from indiscriminate use of firearms, or from exotic infections as from the Ebola or Corona virus. Discussions of average lifespan should, in fact, be replaced by consideration of "median" lifespan – the lifespan of the majority of people, and has that really increased by a decade or two during the past few hundred years?

Back in 44 BC, a Roman senator by the name of Marcus Tullius Cicero wrote a book on aging he called "How to Grow Old." The book was gifted to me by professor Joseph Hofbeck who was responsible for the French translation as well as the title of my last book "Zen in Action." Cicero alludes to Plato who was 81 when he died and Socrates, who was 69 when he was induced to drink the deadly hemlock. Cicero himself was 68 when he wrote the book and refers to many friends who were in their 70's, 80's or 90's when they died. Cicero himself died of assassination at age 69. The three secrets to a long life, Cicero claimed were "to stretch the muscles, exercise the mind, and cultivate a garden." Damn good advice, as valid today as it was centuries ago.

CHAPTER TWO

Theories of Aging

A number of clever people have pondered how and why people age and die. Experts in the field fall roughly into one of two camps: those who believe that aging should be regarded as a natural biological process, fulfilling Darwinian or neo-Darwinian principles and unlikely to be altered by any man-made measures. Then there are those who believe that aging should be regarded as a disease process that can be altered by potions, chemicals or changes in behavior.

The speculations themselves are known as "theories of aging." Some of these speculations have led to further experiments and to studies that have advanced our understanding of the processes involved and to suggestions on how we might add healthy years to our lives. Others have led to dead ends.

Experts who have examined this question looked at the problem from various standpoints. Could it be related to things ingested, that is, can we consume too much of this or too little of that? Could it relate more to how the body handles the intake, its chemistry, in other words. Can the garbage disposal system of the body be overcome or become dysfunctional with age? Can the accumulation of debris in the cells shorten life as it can the life of those particular cells? Could something in the environment: the air, the soil, or the water be a factor? Is lifespan related to geography? Could the study of our genetic make-up, our DNA, reveal the secrets to a long life? Could the study of what controls the lifespan of other creatures, like laboratory rats and mice, or even a single celled organism, provide clues, if not answers?

Let's examine these ideas, one after another.

The first well established idea blames sugar. Excess glucose, it is claimed, combines with other molecules, or protein in the body, to form what are called "cross-links." When this process occurs in the skin it causes the wrinkling we associate with aging. When it occurs in the brain it forms deposits associated with dementia. The deposits are, in fact, the amyloid or amyloid-like bodies seen in the brain of people with Alzheimer's disease. We do not have a way of seeing these plaques in people while they are alive, but they are obvious findings on an autopsy. Why can we not see these plaques in living subjects when we can "see" cancerous lumps or impaired blood flow elsewhere in the body? Amyloid lumps can grow to be an egg sized or orange sized lump in the kidney and do virtually no harm.

As a urologist I have looked after a number of patients with amyloid lumps in their kidney. Why is the clinical course of someone with an amyloid lump in the kidney so different from the patient with an amyloid-like deposit in the brain? Is it because it is amyloid-like and not really amyloid in the brain? They must be different processes, but what are the differences? Why has there been so little progress in our understanding and management of Alzheimer's disease?

When laboratory animals are fed a glucose restricted diet they live longer. This observation has been made now in numerous experiments on different species of animals including worms, flies, mice, rats, and larger animals. The data is persuasive and in keeping with the observations in human subjects, like the one of native Okinawans who restrict food intake twenty percent (hara hachi-bu or stomach 80%) and are known to have long lives. What is much less clear is how much glucose restriction is necessary to produce a worthwhile result.

Do people who were overweight but managed to lose weight and kept the weight off end up living longer lives than those who failed? Does fasting once a week, or regularly once a month, or for a protracted time once every year make any difference? Does a period of severe restriction or starvation provide benefits over a lifetime? Did Holocaust survivors who were incarcerated and starved end up living long lives? What about allied soldiers imprisoned in Hong Kong who were starved by the Japanese military? Did those who outlived their ordeal and emerged horribly emaciated, but alive, have prolonged lives? Have studies been done? If not, why not?

I think enough data have been collected now to suggest that fasting one day per week or eating two meals a day instead of three is profitable and within our capacity to do it. I am considering it.

The idea that glucose may be worse than fat or animal protein in aging mankind is sometimes described by the acronym, AGES, short for Advanced Glycation End Products which, to my understanding, says much the same thing and nothing much more.

Before we leave the subject of sugar and lifespan, though, let me mention what we were taught about nutrition back in the fifties. We were instructed that food was largely carbohydrate, protein, and fat, with traces of other essential items such as vitamins and minerals, like iron, copper, magnesium, and undoubtedly, a few others. Vitamins were also essential and were either water soluble, like vitamins B and C, or water insoluble, like vitamins A, D and E.

Each gram of carbohydrate or protein produced 5 calories while a gram of fat produced 9 calories. An intake of 3,500 extra calories will put on one extra pound, we were told. Thus, whatever else, ingesting 500 calories less each day should result in a one pound weight loss after one week (500x7=3500). There were many booklets that indicated the amount of calories in different food servings. A slice of bread, for example, was so many calories, with butter and jam, it increased to that much more calories.

I have been guilty of telling friends and patients that by consuming 500 calories less each day they should lose one pound after just one week. Not one friend or patient told me that my suggestion worked. I had thought that they could not cut down, but I know better now. It may be correct to say that a slice of bread is so many calories and that with butter and jam it increased in calories. But, within the gut there are good bacteria, known as pro-biotics, whose action on the food consumed changes the calorie count.

Another "theory" blames accumulated debris. The garbage disposal apparatus at the cellular level in mankind resides in the mitochondria, a structure in the cytoplasm of all cells. When the mitochondria are overwhelmed, as in old age or overuse, the argument goes, the cell dies. If enough cells die, lifespan should be affected. The problem with this hypothesis is that, even if it were true, nothing much can be done about it. Well, that was the case until a recent report suggested that his process could be altered by a newly developed preparation. It's too early yet to know whether such a product will really amount to anything. I suspect this "new" product is not the one and only new proposal. Time will tell.

Another largely discredited theory blames "free radicals." The free radical theory of aging was put forward by the chemist, Denham Harman, back in 1956. When a cell burns sugar to produce energy an unstable product, called a free radical, is created. Free radicals are characterized by unpaired electrons on the outer orbit of the atom or molecule, making them unstable and toxic. Free radicals may promote cancer, diabetes, heart disease, or dementia and shorten life, it was proposed, but the toxic products could be neutralized by antioxidants taken as a pill.

Antioxidants are readily available as vitamin C tablets, vitamin E capsules, or one of many over-the-counter health products, like selenium, glutathione (plentiful in mushroom, by the way), pygnogenol, etc. Large scale studies were launched around the world to see if loading up on antioxidants could lower the risks of developing cancer, dementia, diabetes and even lengthen life. The results were disappointing. If anything, the data seemed to show that cancer was promoted and life shortened, not lengthened by extra anti-oxidants.

One very persuasive study took place in Finland where a double blind study compared supplemental Vitamin E to a placebo on the risk of developing prostate cancer. Those placed on the placebo developed cancer less frequently than those on the anti-oxidant!

Curiously, despite these reports, sales of antioxidants continue briskly around the world to this day. The sales pitch of large corporations can be persuasive even when there is little or no scientific data to back it up.

I must mention, though, that allowing free radicals to run loose in the body is like inviting a wild animal into your living room. It can produce havoc. If taking vitamin C and E can lower the risk of potential havoc and do no harm, why not consider it? Remember when the most celebrated chemist of the day, Linus Pauling, was taking over 20 grams of vitamin C everyday? He thought everybody else should be doing likewise.

Linus Pauling, by the way, was the one who might have uncovered the structure of the DNA had not James Watson and Francis Crick beaten him to it. The story is told in captivating fashion by Watson in his book "The Double Helix" published in 1968. There are people who have criticized the account as caring too much about the glory of priority and not enough about sharing credits with other scientists, like Rosalind Franklin and Maurice Wilkins. In my view the real world of science works the way Watson described it.

The proposal of it all being in the genes deserves further comment. It turns out that when it comes to aging, not many genes are involved, except those that appear to be associated with fertility. Animals with extended period of fertility tend to live long, but there is no established connection of vigorous human fertility with longer lives. The idea that our DNA is programmed to extend the life of the community over the life of an individual is an intriguing proposition. The suggestion comes from Josh Mitteldorf, whose book "Cracking the Aging Code" is a delightful read. His book has certainly broadened my understanding of the aging process.

The Blue Zones

Dan Buettner, writing for the National Geographic magazine as well as a book on the subject has identified five areas in the world where many of the inhabitants live very long lives. These areas were once circled on a map with a blue-ink pen and have since been known as "blue zones." The five areas are:
– The island of Ikaria, Greece
– The island of Okinawa, Japan
– Sardinia, Italy
– Loma Linda, California
– Nicoya Peninsula, Costa Rica

Just a moment! Aren't all five areas close to ocean water? Could that be the reason for the longevity? Can we explore that? Do people who live far away from ocean water have shorter lifespan than those who can feel and see ocean air? It does sound reasonable, does it not? Why don't we launch a study?

Nine healthy lifestyle habits of the inhabitants of these five areas were identified:

1. They walked more.
2. They all claimed a purpose in life.
3. They took measures to reduce stress. (Ikarians took naps, Okinawans contemplated their ancestors, Sardinians enjoyed a happy hour, the Seventh Day Adventists of Loma Linda prayed, and Costa Ricans enjoyed their community.)
4. They ate a largely bean based diet with little or no meat.
5. They did not abstain from alcohol and, in fact, consumed a moderate amount.
6. Okinawans adopted the 80% rule, that is, they stopped eating when 80% full (hara hachi-bu). It was never made clear, though, how the Okinawans recognized when they were four/fifth full.
7. They all socialized a lot.
8. They developed a sense of community.
9. They placed family first.

There is nothing out of the ordinary in all of this. There was no magic potion, no secret food or food additive, no special exercise, nothing at all unique and special identified in the atmosphere. All these communities appeared to be behind the times, unaware or uncaring of the technical advances that permeate the life of present-day city dwellers. In fact, with the arrival of McDonalds and Kentucky fried chicken the life span of the younger inhabitants is shortening, for example, in Okinawa.

It is too bad that nothing magical was found in the soil, vegetation, sea food or atmosphere common to the five sites. There was nothing at all that could be made into a "secret" concoction. In fact, even the established longevity appears to be eroding before our eyes.

Searching for Shangri-La does not appear to be the answer to our question. Can there be a real-life Shangri-La? In James Hilton's novel that was made into a classic film, called "Lost Horizon" a small collection of westerners survive an airplane crash in the Himalayas and end up in a remote community there where the inhabitants do not age. After some time and against all advice the rescued group decide to leave the community taking with them a beautiful native woman who has formed a relationship with one of the western men. On the trip out, she tires, collapses, and when her fallen body is turned over she is dead and looks a century older. I can still remember the collective gasp from the audience at that moment.

The Telomere Story

Is it not remarkable that a young woman from Australia, working as a post-doctorate fellow at Yale university could study the chromosomes of a single celled organism living in fresh water ponds, called tetrahymena, and discover how its life, (and thus, presumably, all life) comes to an end? And yet, that is exactly what Elizabeth Blackburn did.

What Blackburn discovered were structures of known chemical composition at the ends of chromosomes, called telomeres, which shortened with each division so that after about forty cell divisions the life of that cell came to an end. Furthermore, Blackburn, along with Carol Greider discovered an enzyme, they named telomerase which stopped the shortening process and, thus, presumably lengthened life. And, in conjunction with another scientist, Elissa Epel, the two women determined that a telomere lengthening process can be brought about by behavioral changes, like meditation. And if meditation can lengthen telomeres so might exercise, proper diet, positive attitude, and having good friends. These studies are presumably underway.

Telomere lengths can be measured, even commercially, from sputum or from white blood cells. I gather that telomeres cannot be long in sputum and short in white blood cells or visa versa. Longer telomeres are associated with longer life and better health, while shorter telomeres are associated with increased risks of heart disease, diabetes, cancer, dementia, and shorter lives.

The telomere story is far from being completely told. The fact that behavioral changes (meditation) can alter telomere length and, thus, lifespan appears indisputable. This finding belies the long-established dogma that acquired characteristics cannot be passed on to the next generation. Telomere length can be measured so then, associations to longer telomeres can be better understood.

One example is the moon of fingernails: the bigger the moon, the longer the telomere. There are studies that show longer telomeres in people who meditate, diet, exercise, or think positively. What I would like to see is a study that measures telomeres before any meditation and then after a period of meditation in the same subjects. Did meditation lengthen the telomere or show only that meditators had longer telomeres to begin with? From my readings so far, I have difficulty answering this critical question. The study of longer lives with longer telomeres was made, after all, by looking at stored blood samples collected decades earlier.

There is one study by Dean Ornish, out of San Francisco, worth relating. He studied men with low grade prostate cancer. The subjects were placed on a diet high in plants and low in fat;

and a regime that involved a thirty minute walk six days every week, yoga stretches, and meditation. After three months, their telomerase increased and stayed increased for the length of the study, which was five years. Is that significant? Men with low grade prostate cancer have, at most, a thirty percent chance of progression, overall. Bottom line – we need more studies!

Veganism

A couple with whom I often played tennis (Shawn and Aisha Moscovitch), introduced me to veganism and to Colin Campbell's book: "The China Study." One cannot read this book without seriously considering "veganism" as a way of life. On principle, vegans will not eat animal- based food, thus excluding not only beef, fish, and fowl, but also milk, cheese and other animal products from their diet. They live on an exclusively plant- based diet, getting their protein largely from soybeans and nuts. They do not look under-nourished and, in fact, are known to live longer and are less susceptible to heart ailments, colorectal cancer, as well as breast and prostate cancer. They are less susceptible to diabetes and dementia as well.

If our only purpose in life was to live as long as possible we must all become vegans. I am willing to sacrifice a few days of my life, though, so that I can enjoy the occasional steak, chicken, or fish. I am willing to cut down on my total intake of animal protein, although it is unlikely that such a move would make an iota of difference. I might be persuaded to cut out animal-based food if I can be promised extra years, but I am certain that such a promise cannot be made. Still, meatless burgers are catching on. There are people who claim they can instantly tell the difference, but I cannot. If meatless burgers are healthier and in the same price range, I am willing to make the switch.

I am less comfortable with Campbell's contention in the

book that the medical profession, cattle and pork lobby, and the giant pharmaceutical firms conspire to keep the public from data harmful to their industry. This is a widely held perception – that if an inexpensive product that can wipe out a killer disease were to be discovered or developed and, if it competed with a popular pharmaceutical product, it will be kept off the shelf to protect an industry thriving because of the problem disease. That view is a little too cynical for me.

If science were to eliminate mosquitos from the face of this planet, for example, I cannot think of a single negative consequence. If they are a feed for fish, I believe fish will survive or can be made to survive without them. We will wipe out malaria, and now the Zita virus as well. I think we can live without mosquitos. We can live as well without the spirochete that causes syphilis, or the virus that causes AIDS, or a pandemic, like Covid-19. But the same cannot be said about other insects, like bees. Without the pollination carried out by bees we would not have the plant life necessary for our very survival. It is an alarming fact that the bee population is dwindling before our eyes. Science has deliberately eliminated smallpox and poliomyelitis and we have not suffered any negative consequences as far as I can tell. There are people who respect the sanctity of life in every living creature but, for me, that is going too far. There are misinformed media personalities, on the other hand, who try to mislead the public about the danger and potential harm of vaccinations.

Why this is permitted baffles me. After all, our society would not allow someone to campaign against defying traffic lights or speed limits. Shouldn't one have a medical degree to dispense medical advice?

So much for theories of aging. There is a lot we know and a lot more we don't know. Enough data has been gathered though, to make some strong recommendations. We should be much more careful about our sugar intake. Excess sugar is the biggest poison we are putting into our bodies to-day. It has replaced the cigarette as our greatest villain. We should consider fasting. One day of fasting per week seems reasonable and doable. Active exercise for 30 minutes daily seems reasonable and doable as well. The argument for meditation is irrefutable. The same applies for yoga.

My personal plan is to combine the three and do it on a regular basis.

I will do ten yoga stretching exercises on my mat. I will try or learn to meditate while I do it. If the process takes less than half an hour, I will simply repeat it. I have just started this but by the time this book project is completed, I should be able to report how successful (or unsuccessful) I have been. I do not like failures!

Here, then, is a link to stretching exercises jooh.no/web/taabs/Flexibility_Ebook_mg.pdf and below is my version:

Without bending knees, touch the toes. At least, get as close as you can to the toes. Keep doing that until the timer indicates you have been trying it for one minute.

1. Place one foot on a step or a chair. Lean forward so that you can feel the muscles on the back below the knees being stretched. Switch to the other foot and keep it up for one minute.
2. Swing your arms, outstretched to the left and to the right. Keep it up for one minute.
3. Sit on a cushion, bend both legs at the knees so that the heels will be touching or almost touching the genitals. With your arms slowly push down the knees towards the ground. Relax, then repeat pushing down the knees, again and again for one minute.
4. Get down on your knees on the yoga mat. Bring the left

foot forward so that it forms a right angle at the knee. Slide the right leg back as much as you can. Repeat, reversing the legs. Continue one minute.

5. Start as in 5, but after the right leg is back, put your hands behind your head and twist your body so that the right elbow swings past the left leg. Switch legs and keep repeating for one minute.

6. Assume position as for push-ups. Keep the hips on the ground, hands by the sides, and look up to the ceiling. Hold and repeat. Continue one minute.

7. Start with the back on the mat and the hands at the sides. The feet are a shoulder width apart. Lift the hips to the sky and bring the hands underneath. Try to bring the chest to the right hand under the chin. Relax and repeat for one minute.

8. Lie on your back. Bring the bent right leg to the chest and hold for 5 seconds. Put arms out to your sides. Twist your body to the left. Repeat reversing legs and carry on for one minute.

9. Lie on your back, knees bent, feet on the ground. Place right ankle on left thigh. Reach between the legs and grab the back of the left leg with the right hand. Grab the other side of the left leg with the left hand. Pull the left leg towards you. Switch legs and continue for one minute.

10. My plan is to make these exercises so routine that I will be able to do them without having to think about what I should be doing next. I have not reached that point, yet. When I do, and I am certain I can get there, I will direct my mind to consider other things. Is that not a stage or form of meditation? I think it is. I hope it is.

Thus, I will meditate, fast, exercise, suppress sugar intake, and start taking metformin. And that should add a decade or more to my lifespan. But, not if I develop a lethal health issue, especially if I don't address it appropriately.

Another question remains: What of the 100 yr. old man who is interviewed and asked "What is your secret to longevity?"

He replies, "Orange juice every morning and pussy every night."

Often these characters who are "larger than life", also admit to eating chocolate bars, drinking alcohol, not exercising (over the course of their lives thus far) and some even smoke cigarettes. How can we justify a prudent life when people who defy it often live very long lives? There will always be exceptions to any rule, especially in the biological sciences. But, these exceptions to the rule, should not detract us from huge population studies, like the one carried out in Formosa. Sedentary people had the shortest lifespan, and it lengthened with more and more physical activity. Just fifteen minutes a day was better than none at all, and with every half hour of added physical activities the lifespan increased in direct correlation.

Now, let us look at the ten most common causes of death in this country and how we might best confront them.

CHAPTER THREE

Lethal Health Issues

I f we were able to live to a ripe old age, let's say into the nineties, and die in our sleep, that is the life that might have been even further extended by diet, exercise, fasting, good friends and good attitude. However, lethal health issues may interrupt our best laid plans. We must examine life threatening health problems because they represent challenges we can, with luck, effort and dedication, overcome to an extent far more than we would normally think possible. I have perused several scholarly books on aging, by recognized and established experts in the field. I have learned a lot, but none of them discuss killing disorders that are shortening lives.

Are they not every bit as important as neo-Darwinian principles that may underlie life span?

It is not difficult to find out what is taking peoples' lives in Canada today. Let us examine the ten most common causes as listed on the internet and derived from reliable sources. We can then discuss what can be done about each one of them, particularly in the more vulnerable senior population. The ten leading causes of death in Canada are reported to be as follows:

1. Cancer
2. Heart disease
3. Strokes
4. Lung disease
5. Accidents

6. Diabetes
7. Alzheimer's disease
8. Influenza and pneumonia
9. Suicide
10. Kidney disease

One: Cancer

A 2017 report from the Canadian Cancer Society indicated that almost fifty percent of Canadians currently alive and over the age of fifty will be diagnosed with cancer in their lifetime and that one in four will die from the disease. The leading killing cancer is still lung cancer, followed by colo-rectal cancer, then prostate cancer in men and breast cancer in women. About two hundred different cancers have been described. Pancreatic cancer and ovarian cancer, for example, though much less common, are frequently fatal because early diagnosis is uncommon. Skin cancers are more obvious even to the naked eye, but it is less well known that two forms, squamous cell carcinoma and melanoma can develop spread sites and take lives, while another form, basal cell carcinoma, can spread locally but not have distant lesions called metastases. Blood, brain, and lymph node cancers may also be less common, but still lethal. Let us examine the common cancers.

LUNG CANCER.

The connection of lung cancer to cigarette smoking is now well established and the deliberate attempt by the cigarette makers to obfuscate this connection has been deliberated in the courts. Cigarette makers have been found guilty and are about to pay for their misdeed. Not all lung cancers, though, are related to cigarette smoking. My good friend and long-time tennis partner, Morrel Bachynski, died of lung cancer and he did not smoke at all. Could he have been saved had I persuaded him to have a chest tomogram earlier when all he had was an annoying cough? Possibly, and I feel guilty I did not encourage him to do so. I would feel more guilty had I been his doctor, but I was his urologist, tennis partner, and friend. Lung cancer comes in two forms: non-small cell and small cell. The latter is more deadly and I suspect that is the form my friend had.

Looking for disease in a healthy individual is known as screening. For lung cancer the recommended screening test consists of three consecutive low dose CT scans of the chest, sometime between the ages of 55 and 74. Screening for lung cancer is certainly more appropriate for those with a family history of lung cancer, as well as for those who smoke or are exposed to second hand smoke, and for those with known exposure to radon and asbestos. Radon is the radioactive gas formed by the decay of naturally occurring uranium-238, and asbestos is the fire-retardant material that can encourage the development of mesothelioma and lung cancer.

Looking for disease after the development of symptoms usually translates into a delayed or late diagnosis. The symptoms associated with lung cancer are persistent cough, chest pain, shortness of breath, weight loss, hoarseness and bronchitis. The presence of these symptoms does not denote the presence of cancer nor do their absence assure freedom from the disease.

Certainly it is a fact that, at this time, the only way we can beat lung cancer is to discourage smoking and to get a routine chest tomogram (CT) regularly so that an early diagnosis will not be missed. Lung cancer can be cured with ablative surgery when the diagnosis is early. We have little to offer when the disease is advanced although more extensive surgery, radiotherapy and chemotherapy in various combinations have helped some patients.

Why do we not do low dose chest tomograms more regularly? Studies that addressed this question revealed that many false positive results occur. That is, the tomogram suggests something is wrong, inviting legitimate alarm, but follow up studies reveal that in over ninety seven percent of the time – there is no cancer! Is that a reason to abandon screening? I don't think so, although not everybody may agree with me! I suspect every person with a late diagnosis wishes he had earlier screening. Might there be a better way to make the early and accurate diagnosis of lung cancer? Has routine sputum cytology ever been looked at as a test to make the early diagnosis? Can it help make an earlier diagnosis? Can an ordinary chest x-ray repeated at regular intervals rule in or rule out early lung cancer as well as the CT scan? Can a diagnosis be made without a biopsy or is biopsy always necessary? Are there toxins in the air other than cigarette smoke that causes lung cancer? Something besides asbestos and radon? What are the real facts about rays we cannot see, like those emitted by microwave ovens, or radio transmissions? Many questions can be asked, but when we still can't get every young person to resist the allure of a cigarette, what's the point of wasting time, money and energy pursuing other villains?

Let me relate a true story. I was the urologist for a successful businessman, originally from Australia. He came to see me once a year to make certain his prostate and genito-urinary system were okay. On his visit one year he said he did not have long to live as he had been diagnosed with advanced lung cancer. I was told to "go home and die," he said, with his macabre brand of what I thought was Australian humor. "Let's, at least, get another opinion," I suggested. I referred him to the highly regarded chief of Surgery and the doctor for the Montreal Canadiens Hockey Team, Dr. David Mulder. David looked at the x-ray and told the patient that it didn't look like cancer to him. Further investigations revealed that what he had was an advanced fungal infection and he was cured with drugs and surgery.

What is the bottom line as far as lung cancer is concerned? Don't smoke, beware of second hand smoke, remain alert about possible toxins in the air, and consider low dose chest tomograms on a regular basis, especially if you have a history of smoking or there is a family history of the disease. Lung cancer is a killing disease: Don't miss out on an opportunity for an early diagnosis and cure. Get the low dose chest tomograms as suggested.

Recently, I lost another good friend to lung cancer, and she was not a smoker as well. I don't doubt that lung cancer is the number one cancer killer!

Can anything be done to reduce the risks? Anything, that is, other than to discourage smoking or exposing the lungs to other toxins? Science should be a little more forthcoming with information. How toxic are car exhausts or industrial smoke? Would we be told if curbing it may damage a thriving industry?

Lung cancer in people who don't smoke, look after their health and watch what they eat seems totally unfair. But then, what is fair or unfair when we are dealing with cancer?

COLO-RECTAL CANCER

Colo-rectal cancer is the number two cancer killer. We can reduce mortality from this cancer by ascertaining routine regular colonoscopies. We cannot make colonoscopies mandatory but, perhaps, we can make the testing of stool for occult blood a more popular test than it is.

Maybe, people can be taught how to do the testing themselves. It does not seem to me unreasonable to ask patients to poke their solid waste with a dipstick and note a color change.

This must be done, of course, after several days abstinence of any iron intake. There are frequent and loud complaints about the long wait for a routine colonoscopy in Canada, but you can be certain that if you asked the loudest complainer if he has ever looked into having his stool tested for occult blood the universal answer is invariably "No".

Can a person have colon or rectal cancer without a trace of blood in his stool? Not likely! The definitive diagnostic test, though, is the colonoscopy. Most people find the preparation, the cleansing and evacuation of the bowel before the examination more trying than the colonoscopy itself.

The colonoscopy would ascertain the presence of colonic polyp(s) which can be removed at the time of the procedure. A polyp, left alone, can become a cancer nine years later. Does that mean that a virtual colonoscopy, an imaging test, is a total waste of time? Not really. A negative virtual colonoscopy can save a person the discomfort of an actual direct examination.

Would a stool examination for the presence of blood obviate the need for a colonoscopy? Not entirely. Furthermore, a colonoscopy can rule in or rule out other disorders of the gastro-intestinal system like Crohn's disease, ulcerative colitis, or diverticulitis. A simple stool test for occult blood cannot do that.

Can we lower the risk of developing colon and rectal cancer by changing our eating habits? There are hints that we can, by taking certain pro-biotics (although I am uncertain of the details) and eating more cruciferous vegetables, like broccoli, cabbage, Swiss chard, cauliflower, bock choy, and Brussel sprout but the evidence is not overwhelming. It's not as if loading up on the protective foods can eliminate the risk. At best it might lower the risk a tiny bit.

When the diagnosis is early, a fairly large segment of bowel with the disease is removed and the shortened bowel rejoined, but when the disease is at or near the rectum that cannot be done and a bag has to be worn over the bowel that is made to end on the abdominal wall. That is known as the colostomy.

Why does colon cancer occur more often in certain families, and why is Crohn's disease so common in the Jewish population? Is it related to genes, diet, or what? At this point we don't know. What can be said for certain is that people who have had an early diagnosis will come out ahead of those whose diagnosis was delayed for one reason or another. Don't quarrel with the recommendation to have the colonoscopy!

So, what's the bottom line as far as colo-rectal cancer is concerned? Don't object to the routine colonoscopy. The frequency of follow-ups will depend upon whether polyps have been seen and removed. Don't quarrel with the recommendation for subsequent follow-ups. A positive family history for colo-rectal cancer may encourage you to consider pro-biotics and more cruciferous vegetables. You may want to consider the two protective products (probiotics and cruciferous vegetables) even without a family history. Remember that early diagnosis means curable disease, usually with no colostomy or limitations in lifestyle. We may not be able to prevent colon cancer from ever occurring at this point, but we can certainly reduce its chances of shortening lives.

PROSTATE CANCER

The third most common killing cancer in men is prostate cancer. If we categorized colon cancer separately from rectal cancer, prostate cancer becomes the number two most frequent cancer killer in men. By far, prostate cancer is the most common cancer in the adult male. The fact that more men die with than from prostate cancer has obfuscated the issue. Well-meaning advice is often skewed: don't bother, stop testing at seventy, complications from invasive testing is worse than doing nothing – all bad counsel as far as I am concerned.

Prostate cancer is a curable cancer, made incurable by a delayed diagnosis. Early on, there are no signs or symptoms. The disease may have been suspected because there is a family history of the disease or the gland may not have felt right on the dreaded rectal examination or the PSA reading might have been abnormal. PSA (prostate specific antigen) is a protein made virtually exclusively by the prostate gland. Elevated readings of this protein or accelerated increase suggest a possibility of this cancer. At one time a PSA reading over 4 was considered suspicious. Today, a more important interpretation of this blood test is an increase of over 0.75 units in one year. The ratio of free to total PSA is also used to select those more likely to have the cancer. When the ratio is over 25%, cancer is unlikely; when the ratio is under 10% the suspicion is high, while most readings are between 10 and 25%. When the blood test or the rectal examination or both tests are out of line, an ultrasound guided transrectal biopsy of the prostate used to be the next step. Today, the appropriate next step is the MRI (magnetic resonance imaging) which can better select the candidates who should be biopsied. The biopsy is guided by the MRI imaging and is thus much more accurate.

Prostate cancer can vary in their severity from those that are unlikely to progress (a Gleason 6 or less) to those of intermediate severity (Gleason 7), to those likely to kill when left alone (Gleason 8-10). The Gleason grade is a score assigned by the pathologist after microscopy. It is named after Donald Gleason, the pathologist who first described and proposed it.

Patients are advised simple monitoring when the biopsy reveals a low-grade cancer (Gleason 6 or less). There is a 30% chance that the disease will progress, as signified by increasing readings of their PSA done every 6 months or more disease on the biopsy also repeated every six or twelve months. There is also a 70% chance that the disease will not progress and will not require any treatment at all. Regular follow ups, though, are mandatory.

When the disease is more aggressive (Gleason 7 or higher), but the PSA is less than 10, the curative treatment is surgical removal of the gland or radiotherapy of one kind or another. As a rule, if the patient is otherwise fit and under seventy years of age, surgery is advised over radiotherapy because any patient who fails to be cured by surgery can have radiotherapy but surgery is not a legitimate option after failure of radiotherapy. That is because the complication rate of the surgery becomes unacceptably high.

Radiated tissue does not heal as well as non-radiated tissue. When the cancer is already spread beyond the prostate gland, as signified by a positive bone scan, or suggested by high PSA readings and enlarged lymph nodes in the pelvis on the CT scan, different forms of hormone therapy and chemotherapy are utilized. The treatment, obviously, is not always successful in terms of a permanent control, but there is almost always a successful immediate response to treatment. Sometimes, the disease stays controlled for decades, at other times for years, and sometimes, only for months. Recently the results of hormone therapy have been further improved by the development of two new hormone controlling drugs.

Let me make two more points before we leave the subject of prostate cancer.

About a half a century ago, there was an interesting study done, I think, in Britain. As early prostate cancer can be symptom free, and as these patients were often elderly, could early administration of hormone therapy be doing more harm than good? The doctors who did the study discovered that men who had early treatment fared far better – their time to more disease and time to death was significantly better than those whose treatment began only when they became symptomatic from the disease.

Secondly, it used to be thought that different ways to eliminate testosterone from the male body, that is, by surgical castration, by the administration of estrogens or by drugs that instructed the master gland of the body, the pituitary, to stop the testicles from producing testosterone did not differ in their efficacy in fighting the disease. Not so! Furthermore, drugs recently developed that interfere with testosterone production at different points in their production, like Abiraterone or Enzalutimide, can be effective therapy in patients failing the traditional testosterone eliminating therapy, widely known as androgen deprivation therapy. I suspect that the time may come when we use different combinations of the various preparations, cycling them to best advantage.

I have spent a significant part of my life looking after men with prostate cancer. I am impressed with the enormous progress made in my professional lifetime. I no longer see the hospital beds filled with men with advanced prostate cancer in severe pain and distress. Nevertheless, we can always do better.

Can we prevent the cancer from ever developing? There are hints that we may be able to do so. This common cancer in the western world is much less common in Japanese men living in Japan. But, when the Japanese men emigrate to North America and have lived in America for more than ten years they develop prostate cancer just as frequently as the white man. Prostate cancer is also known to be more common in the black population.

When people emigrate, their genes do not change. What may

change is diet and lifestyle. Obviously, the study that needs to be done is to determine the incidence of prostate cancer in white men who have lived in Japan for more than ten years. Is their incidence of prostate cancer less? Can that be related to dietary changes? I have tried to initiate this study several times without success.

Screening for prostate cancer will undoubtedly lower the death rate from prostate cancer. Furthermore, I don't think the screening should stop at seventy as commonly recommended. I used to tell patients whose family doctor stopped PSA testing at seventy to go back to their doctor and ask him or her when he was going to die because stopping the screening presumed the doctor knew.

The recommendation is based on the recognized lifespan of the population but, just because the average life-span in the country is 85, that does not mean the particular candidate will not live to be 95. Why any sentient being would shun the screening tests; a rectal exam and the PSA blood test once a year, baffles me but I know a number of men, including urologists, who choose not to be screened. Semen changes with the onset of prostate cancer is an interesting question. Why can't a medical student or a resident be assigned to explore this question?

BREAST CANCER AND OVARIAN CANCER

After lung and colorectal cancer, the most common killing cancer in women is breast cancer.

Breast cancer is the most common cancer in women just as prostate cancer is the most common cancer in men. Is it not interesting that both cancers occur in glands that are vestigial (no obvious presence or microscopic) in childhood and develop only after puberty? The size, shape and form of the female breast has fascinated mankind from time immemorial. Artists have capitalized on this fascination. Why malignancies develop so commonly in this tissue has never been explained. The genetic aspect of this malignancy has been elucidated to some extent. Women with a defective BRC1 or BRC2 gene, which normally fix damaged cells, become more likely to develop breast cancer (an increase from 12% to 80%) or ovarian cancer (where the increased risk is 40% from 1.3% in those with this specific genetic disorder.) Men with this gene disorder increase their risk for developing prostate cancer as well but I am unaware of the comparable figures for men.

Some prominent personalities, like Angelina Jolie, chose to have her breasts and ovaries removed after proving positive for the gene. Whether that should be done for everybody who tests positive remains controversial.

Breast cancer screening attempts to make an earlier diagnosis of the disease. In addition to asking women to check themselves for the presence of an abnormal lump on a monthly basis, and to look for changes, like the puckering of the skin, changes in the shape or appearance of the breasts in front of a mirror - an x-ray test of the breast called a mammogram is advised every 2 to 3 years between the ages of 50 to 69. There is little radiation from a breast mammogram. Women declining the test for fear of test related complications are making a mistake. Women found to have an abnormality in the mammogram are instructed to have an ultrasound examination of the breasts. Then, with persistent suspicion, a needle or open biopsy of the suspicious area will have to be done. Like all cancers, outcome will depend upon the aggressive nature of the cancer, the extent of the disease, and the response to the treatment.

To-day the accepted treatment for the early diagnosis of breast cancer is the surgical removal of the lump (lumpectomy) followed by a course of radiotherapy. It is an interesting fact that it took a very long time; decades, in fact, to prove that this way of treating the disease produced far better results than by carrying out a mutilating procedure that removed the entire breast along with the draining lymph nodes in the axilla. That procedure left many women disfigured with a high probability of significant swelling of the arm on the affected side.

When the disease is already widely spread at the time of diagnosis, though, a combination of chemotherapy and radiotherapy is considered but successful outcomes are infrequent.

Early in my professional career, during the sixties and seventies, I was, at times, asked by female patients to check their breasts because they thought they could feel a lump. I did not hesitate to carry out the examination. After the seventies, though, I hesitated acceding to these requests and certainly not without the presence of a clinic nurse. Doctors could be accused of sexual misdemeanor and, without the presence of a nurse, there was no defense should such a charge be made. It is a sad commentary on our modern life.

Ovarian cancer is even more enigmatic as there are no acknowledged screening tests. Early disease is difficult to diagnose because there are no early symptoms or signs. The symptoms commonly associated with the disease, like feeling bloated, having pain in the pelvis, feeling full or having indigestion, or frequent urination, are all not specific enough to help an early diagnosis. Late diagnosis can be lethal.

The early diagnosis is usually made accidentally, when an ultrasound or CT test of the lower abdomen is done for other reasons. Why should an ultrasound examination for screening purposes not be done then on a regular basis, like once a year? Genetic testing for the BRC1 and BRC2 gene alteration is certainly worthwhile. Women who test positive for the gene alteration increase their risk of developing ovarian cancer from 1.3%

to 40%. Let me repeat that. Women have a 1.3 percent chance of developing ovarian cancer overall, but if positive for the BRC1 or BRC2 gene change the risk becomes 40 percent. It is no wonder then that prophylactic removal of breasts and ovaries is a serious consideration when the gene test is positive. Angelina Jolie, who had a family history and who tested positive chose to have both breasts and ovaries removed as indicated earlier. It remains controversial and uncertain whether such action should become the routine. Chemotherapy for advanced ovarian cancer has helped several patients and is worth a consideration. When the disease is widespread, though, it is debatable whether as much harm can be done as good.

Should every woman, then, with or without a family history have gene testing and an annual ultrasound to ascertain ovarian health? Perhaps! Any harm in doing that? Not that I can think of, other than the cost and the inconvenience.

OTHER LETHAL CANCERS

There are a number of other killing cancers that affect mankind. They include brain cancers, skin cancers (melanoma and squamous cell cancer), uterine and cervical cancers, blood cancers (leukemia), lymph node cancers (lymphoma), pancreatic cancer, thyroid cancer, and bone cancers to name the more common ones. In fact, almost any part of the human body can become an initial site of a malignancy, and about two hundred serious cancers are recognized.

It is widely believed that the threat of cancer is always present and held in check by a protective immune system. Clinical disease occurs according to this thesis when the immune system cannot overcome the initial insult. Current research is concentrating on aiding and stimulating the immune system to better cope with the problem. Cancer immunotherapy is also making progress. The immune cells, or T-cells, exposed to the cancer cells are grown in vats outside the body and injected back into the patient. Such treatments are already underway to treat prostate cancer, as an example, with encouraging results. We are on the threshold of major advances.

It might be noted as well that the immune system is not a totally involuntary system. It can be turned on with laughter and turned off with despair. An optimist, in other words, may come out ahead of a pessimist as far as fighting cancer is concerned. Somewhat like lengthening telomeres, we might be in more control of our destiny than we think. Health care professionals must consider treating not just the physical body but the psychological and immunological well-being of their patients as well.

Without scratching my head too much I can think of far too many people close to me who have lost their life to cancer.

My father died of stomach cancer. An earlier diagnosis was missed because the original barium meal x-ray done on suspicion by the family doctor was erroneously read and by the time a gastroscopy was done, the cancer was advanced and widespread. He had surgery just to unblock an obstruction and chemotherapy was tried but it was the missed early diagnosis that took his life. My father had lived a full and productive life and never complained.

Acute leukemia claimed the life of two good friends. One was a diamond expert, a father of two doctor sons, and the person who got me to play tennis, which added to my life and health. I played with him regularly up to a week before he died. He had a galloping form of the disease which claimed his life within days of the diagnosis.

The other was a good friend who was my classmate in my first year of high school. He responded dramatically to the initial treatment, which included Gleevac, but when the disease returned, nothing worked.

Melanoma claimed the life of an Ear Nose and Throat surgeon, who was two years behind me in schooling.

Prostate cancer took the life of two urologists who were my colleagues. One of them had widespread metastatic disease at the time of diagnosis. He had looked after numerous patients with prostate cancer but, obviously, never bothered with his own health.

Another colleague, three years my junior, died of brain cancer. He was a good friend, ahead of his time in computer expertise, and he had planned our future together. "When we get older, he said, "we will practice together as one specialist. That way, we will only work half as much and enjoy our senior years twice as much more." Unfortunately, that never happened.

Cancer will continue to claim lives, but progress in earlier diagnosis and better drugs and treatments are also having an impact. I believe we are winning the war on cancer.

Here then is my last word on cancer. We can reduce our risk of developing the disease by eliminating our exposure to recognized carcinogens, like cigarette, oriental pickles, unnecessary radiation, certain viruses, like condyloma accuminata or become immunized against it (Gardisil), make certain opportunity for the earlier diagnosis is not missed (get screened), watch out for the latest news on genes and their modifications. We should continue to increase our awareness of DNA manipulations but not become preoccupied with it.

Many cancers can be cured when the diagnosis is early. Don't miss out on that by declining screening tests. We used to think of cancer as an inevitably fatal disease. Today cancer is looked upon more and more as a chronic illness.

I think that cancer as a cause of death will continue to decline particularly in populations aware of screening, pre and pro-biotics (an emerging field of which I know very little) and advances in immunotherapy and stem cell therapy. Cancer should no longer be viewed as an inevitably fatal disease but rather more as a chronic illness. Furthermore, preventative measures, such as reducing exposure to known carcinogens, assuring early diagnosis and curative treatments will all lessen the odds of having lifespan shortened by the number one cause of a premature and untimely demise.

Two: Heart Disease

Whenever there is mention of heart disease, many people think automatically about heart attacks, technically known in medicine as "myocardial infarction." This means that there has been a rather sudden blockage in the arterial blood flow to the heart muscles resulting in death of the muscle cells supplied by that particular artery. When the blockage is significant the attack is incompatible with life. The "attack" is more likely to occur in an artery already damaged by cholesterol deposits. It makes sense, then, for the vulnerable population, like older men and women, to lower the risks of heart attacks by thinning the blood with medications like heparin, Coumadin, Plavix, Eliquis, Pradaxa, Xarelto, Aspirin, or any other competing blood thinning medications. Cholesterol lowering drugs, like Lipitor, Ezetrol, Crestor etc. can also be helpful in lowering the risks. Most people tolerate these pills well, but the occasional patient may have disturbing side effects. The decision, then, to take the pills can become difficult. Cholesterol levels are checked in people who have been fasting and the most important reading is the level of the bad cholesterol, called LDL cholesterol. The ideal reading is under 2.5 or 3.0, and such a level can be reached or approached by taking pills, like Lipitor, often combined with another pill called Ezetrol, or similar competing regimes. Obviously, cutting down on fat rich foods, like beef and dairy fat must also be part of the consideration.

The problem in real life is that heart problems are hardly ever black or white. A serious heart attack may be commonly associated with a crushing chest pain, but attacks just as serious may cause only an unexplained left shoulder tip pain, discomfort in the jaws, an indigestion, or no symptoms at all. In fact, when the blockage is in the main left descending artery, there is usually a sudden death, nothing else. For this reason, disease in this vessel is often called the "widow maker."

Let me relate a personal story.

While vacationing in Florida with my oldest daughter and her family I experienced a heaviness in my left arm playing tennis. I thought little of it because the symptom was not severe. My daughter insisted that I consult a cardiologist upon our return. I promised. Upon my return I played tennis again as was my custom.

"If I develop heaviness in my arm I will have to retire," I said to my partner.

"Of course!" said my friend.

Moments after I began to play the heaviness was back. I decided to give it another minute before I retired. However, the heaviness was gone and did not return at all even after a full hour of play. If the heaviness was from the heart, it should have persisted or worsened, I thought.

But a promise is a promise so I called the cardiologist.

"Drop whatever you are doing and come and see me immediately," the cardiologist, Dr. Allan Sniderman, said to me.

I had a cardiogram which was normal, then a stress cardiogram.

"The heaviness is back," I said.

Allan rushed over to see the tracing.

"You're not leaving," he said. "I will arrange an immediate angiogram."

I had significant blockages in three spots. The worst, I think, was in the left descending artery – the widow-maker!

I had a triple by-pass performed by cardiac surgeon, Dr. Benoit De Varennes, and his team, and I have been perfectly healthy ever since, now more than ten years later. In fact, I no longer have attacks of indigestion which, I suspect, was a masquerading cardiac symptom.

Like every other patient booked for a by-pass operation I was visited by a resident-in-training the night before my operation.

"I have to tell you that there is a 3% chance of mortality associated with this operation," he said.

"Wow! When we do a radical prostatectomy, we tell the patient there is a 1% chance of mortality," I said.

I have found out since that the mortality risk for a by-pass operation is closer to 5%. The risk of dying is significantly less for a stent placement, but the long-term results are much better for the by-pass as long as you survive it. When I was hospitalized, I was under the care of Dr. Nadia Giannetti and after discharge, I came under the care of Dr. Magdi Sami, who continues to look after me. I am grateful for their expert care.

Cardiac revascularization has a Montreal aside to the story. Let me relate it. Doctor Arthur Vineberg was a general surgeon long interested in a surgical answer to victims of heart attacks. He determined that unlike any other organ or tissue in the body, blood flow to the heart could be augmented by inserting an extra vessel directly into the heart muscle. Anywhere else, into any other muscle of the body and the blood flow will stop where the inserted vessel ends and blood does not enter the muscle but, in the heart, the added flow is accepted by the unique nature of heart muscles. The internal mammary artery, which lies close by and which is not essential for normal life could be dissected out of its normal position and inserted into the heart muscle. It worked!

The procedure was supplanted by the by-pass procedure wherein a vein graft obtained from the leg or the same internal mammary artery or a vessel harvested from elsewhere, like the internal iliac artery, or even a synthetic Dacron graft is stitched from a normal vessel to a point in the cardiac artery beyond the area of blockage, by-passing it.

I started my internship in Surgery with Dr. Vineberg in 1960. I ended up becoming his urologist.

Heart disease, though, is not just coronary artery problems. We can have heart disorders from birth, called congenital heart disease. We can also have valve problems, pericardial problems, and heartbeat problems. I remember looking after a patient during my internship. He had a viral infection of the pericardium, which is like an apron over the heart. He didn't feel sick and wondered why he had to be in hospital. Within a week or two, he was dead. Heart valve problems used to be much more common before the introduction of Penicillin, as it was one of the complications of rheumatic fever. Aortic valve disorder is quite common in the senior population to-day, but it is not necessarily progressive and life-threatening. Irregular heartbeat is also common but seldom life threatening. In fact, it is almost unheard of to live to a ripe age without some irregularity of the heartbeat. Cardiologists will manipulate a combination of drugs to keep the senior citizen alive and well as they have done for me.

My wife once asked me whether a portable defibrillator was on hand at the tennis club where I played. I found it that there was one onsite but was uncertain as to whether the staff knew how to deploy it.

Many, many disorders are associated with the heart. That is

why we have cardiologists, who are experts of heart disease, and cardiac surgeons, who are surgeons of heart disorders. Between them, they keep our hearts beating much longer than if nothing was done. As patients we respect and honor them as we should. They are not all perfect though. I know a highly skilled, superb cardiac surgeon who is a chain-smoker. Baffling!

Bottom line: Keep cardiac issues to a minimum by ascertaining that the LDL cholesterol is not abnormally high. Change lifestyle and diet, consider blood thinners and cholesterol lowering drugs if the levels are abnormally high. Regular cardiograms and visits to the cardiologist must become routine once we are past middle age. But don't let preoccupation with your heart run your life. Always keep two baby aspirins in your wallet or purse, just in case! The instruction from the experts is to chew the two baby aspirins and swallow before considering anything else!

With my personal history of a triple by-pass more than ten years ago I couldn't help but wonder if vigorous activity, like tennis, is still good for me. I have been assured by the experts to carry on. "Keep active!" they tell me, so I will! I have enjoyed working on this manuscript, so I will continue that as well as the tennis and golf. I am also old-fashioned in my reading habits, preferring books to screens.

Heart disease may be the number two killer of mankind. At the same time consider how resilient this organ really is. How often have you heard of people dropping dead because their heart stopped beating? It can happen, certainly, but it is not a common occurrence. It occurs in the elderly, often during sleep – I can think of no better way to go! Have you heard of anyone, male or female, perhaps a hundred years old, who died suddenly because his or her heart stopped beating? I suppose it can happen, but it is certainly not a common occurrence.

Can you imagine building a pump that delivers a pulsatile

force of fluid sixty to eighty times a minute that is built to last a century or more? Isn't it curious that we didn't know that that is what the heart does until William Harvey first proposed it about four hundred years ago?

I suspect we already had sharp swords that could sever limbs four hundred years ago. It should have been obvious that when thick walled vessels are cut blood spurts out under pressure and when thin walled vessels are severed blood oozes out. Furthermore, traffic in the thin walled vessels is always in the direction of the heart as can be demonstrated by dangling your arm, see the surface vessels or veins distend with blood; push the flow towards the heart and it can be done with ease: push the flow in the opposite direction and the one way traffic is ascertained by valves within the thin walled vessels. Try it and see for yourself.

Should William Harvey be allowed to return to us today, what would surprise him the most? Would it be the fact that we could restart a heart that has stopped beating by compressing the rib cage repeatedly, that is, by applying external cardiac massage? Would he be more impressed by our ability to pass a metallic stent from inside an artery in the axilla to stent a blockage within a vessel in the heart? Or, would he be more impressed that we could substitute heart function with an external device or heart-lung machine while we fix what is broken within the heart, and expect the heart to resume its function after the repair? I think he would be surprised at what mankind has achieved. Too bad we spend so much of our time and energy trying to take and shorten lives instead of working to improve and extend it.

Three: Stroke

Strokes, medically called CVA (for cardiovascular accidents), means a bleed or a blockage of an artery going to the brain. As we all know, a massive accident causes instant death and a lesser one will be associated with paralysis of a limb or, an inability to speak, or a loss of one function or another depending upon the area of the brain that has been affected. A bleed is more likely to occur in someone with an elevated blood pressure, and blockage more often in someone with more cholesterol build-up in the arteries. Thus, preventative measures will focus on lowering the blood pressure or thinning the blood and often both. The two types of strokes, a bleed or a blockage occur with equal frequency. If we had to choose just one helpful preparation for this disorder at the moment of crisis, that one drug will be Aspirin. Chew two baby Aspirins before considering anything else at the onset of trouble, the popular adage goes. Wise counsel, to be sure.

Strokes will occur more often in the senior citizen as aged blood vessels are more likely to bleed or block. Also, a catastrophic stroke will occur more often at or after a celebration of some kind because a break from the usual routine places extra stresses on an already fragile vasculature.

The blood flow to the brain comes from arteries in the neck called the carotid artery – one left and the other right. These two arteries pulsate in the neck and can be felt by an examining finger. The health of the flow can also be checked with a dye injection called an angiogram as is done for testing blood flow to the heart or other organs. Oddly enough, though, it is controversial whether an apparent blockage in the carotid artery, complete or incomplete, should be surgically fixed or not. It seems logical to fix the blockage, but there is no overwhelming evidence that it helps! It is all together bizarre.

The will to live is powerful and I continue to be impressed with senior citizens who have survived a massive stroke and, despite serious limitations of their cognitive as well as their physical capacities, welcome the daily challenges of life. We should introduce these hardy souls to people with sound physical bodies contemplating ending their lives. I suspect these patients may change the minds of many of them.

Bottom line: What, then, should a person do to minimize his risk of having his life shortened by a stroke? The answer is quite simple. He must keep his blood pressure from climbing too high and he must counteract degenerative changes to his blood vessels. As a bleed or a blockage in the artery to the brain occur with equal frequency and prophylactic measures are the same as those for diseases of the coronary blood vessels: medications to lower blood pressure and pills to thin the blood. Everyone beyond middle age should have two baby aspirin tablets on them just in case.

I am surprised I do not have much more to say about strokes. Among people I know, though, strokes seemed always to have occurred at or after a celebration of some kind, like a birthday party, a reunion, or a holiday trip. Life without celebration seems silly, but a stroke is too heavy a price to pay for a pleasure that is momentary.

Four: Lung Disease

The fourth most common cause of death in Canada is listed as lung disease. As lung cancer has already been discussed as the most common killing cancer and as Influenza and Pneumonia are listed together as the eighth most frequent killer, what are the lung diseases that are being implicated here? They must be asthma, chronic obstructive pulmonary disease (COPD), bronchiectasis, pulmonary embolism and pulmonary fibrosis.

Asthma seldom starts in the senior citizen. But, that is changing. It is not unheard of to-day for people in their eighties to develop asthma for the first time in their life. It has happened to me! At the age of 83, without a background of allergies, lung issues, or smoking, I started to cough incessantly. My internist had a chest x-ray done which was negative and sent me to a lung specialist. He diagnosed asthma right away which was confirmed, I gather, by breathing tests and sputum tests. I was miserable until hefty doses of prednisone made me comfortable. I am now off the prednisone but taking an inhaler called Breo (corticosteroid and bronchodilator), and a biologic medication taken as a bimonthly injection, called Fasenra. I don't cough as much and I can breathe better, but my nose gets plugged from time to time. I am back on Nasonex from time to time which was first suggested to me by a family doctor at the clinic where I used to work.

Asthma can be a life threatening or even life ending problem in children and in young adults. I suspect that is true for the elderly as well. The afflicted individual can breathe in but breathing out is often made more difficult by spasm of the muscles of the breathing tubes and inflammation in the tissue surrounding them. Many drugs, taken by mouth or as a spray, have been developed to reverse the problem but, unfortunately, they do not all always work.

The muscles surrounding the breathing tubes become overactive constricting the passage making breathing out more difficult. There is also associated inflammation of the tissue. Medications can counteract the excess contraction of the muscles that are constricting the passage. When the disease is severe, cortisone-type pills are used to counteract the excess inflammation. As asthma is a kind of overreaction of the body to an insult, medications to suppress the body's over-reaction have been developed, like Nucala and Fasenra, with very worthwhile results as has been the case with me.

Chronic obstructive pulmonary disease is not a Pediatric disorder. It occurs in older adults, particularly if their lungs have been insulted and damaged by long-term cigarette smoking, or by exposure to toxins in the air. It seems reasonable to suspect that such compromised lungs would be more likely to succumb to pneumonia or pneumonia-like disorders. That has proven to be true.

In bronchiectasis, the delicate breathing tubes called bronchi will have become abnormally widened and cannot function to take in oxygen and blow off carbon dioxide as they normally should. Imagine the breathing unit to be like a balloon, expanding on breathing in and deflating on breathing out. An old balloon that is permanently overstretched, inflated or not, is like the lung of a person with bronchiectasis. Such lungs, as in the case of COPD (chronic obstructive pulmonary disease) cannot make gas exchanges adequately and will be more vulnerable to attacks from bacteria and viruses. That, of course, is pneumonia.

Pulmonary embolism means that a blood clot that has formed in a vein of a leg or in the pelvis has migrated to the lung. A large clot will cause a sudden, instant death. A shower of tiny clots will produce an illness not unlike a pneumonia. The risk of pulmonary embolism is heightened by prolonged immobilization, like a long airplane flight. Blood thinning medications, active mobilization and support hose can all reduce the risks. When you are on a trip to a distant location, it would be wise to incorporate support hose, aspirin, and a vigorous walk up and down the airplane aisle as part of your regime. Adoption of such a preventative regime can be a lifesaver.

Pulmonary fibrosis, a kind of scarring of lung tissue, is an exceedingly rare disorder. Often, the cause cannot be determined. Certain drugs, like nitrofurantoin, are associated with this very rare side effect. In fact, as this complication is so uncommon and as the benefits of a medication, like nitrofurantoin, so worthwhile, there is little or no hesitation by doctors to prescribe the drug. Nevertheless, once the diagnosis of pulmonary fibrosis is ascertained, and the offending drug stopped, there is usually no life-threatening progressive damage to the lungs but the damage already done is largely irreversible. More often, though, pulmonary fibrosis occurs without an identifiable culprit.

Lungs are delicate tissue, and unnecessary exposure to toxic chemicals, like tobacco or asbestos, or toxins released into the atmosphere is downright criminal with the knowledge that has been accumulated.

Can anything be done to reduce the chances of having life shortened by these lung diseases? Lungs are delicate tissue deserving of our respect. Insulting them with cigarette smoke or similar noxious chemicals, even marijuana, vaping, or unseen rays is one step away from a suicidal behavior as far as I am concerned. In 2018, Canada has condoned the release of marijuana for public consumption. I am not convinced that it is as safe and innocuous as made out to be. I hope I am wrong. Quebec politicians have decided to raise the permissible age for the consumption of marijuana from eighteen to twenty-one. Their stance should be applauded.

Bottom line: Isn't it fascinating that as we gain more and better control of certain toxins, such as cigarettes and asbestos, we are tempted to try other products in its place, like marijuana or whatever it is that is in "vaping"? Is it not enough that we have recognized toxins we can ill control?

Five: Accidents

Fatal accidents are listed as the fifth most common cause of death in this country. Mishaps can occur at any age, but the frail elderly are at higher risks for life-taking accidents compared to younger adults or children. Falling out of bed and breaking a hip may be the arch prototype, but other accidents, like slipping on the curb, falling on stairways, or slipping on ice are all common occurrences. All accidents, in retrospect, are damn-right ridiculous and foolish. We can laugh about it most of the time. But, not always! Serious accidents will continue to occur because the alternative, staying inactive, might be even worse.

Perhaps it is important to distinguish serious life-threatening accidents, like a head-on car collision from less serious incidents which can, nevertheless, lead to lifestyle changes that shortens lives. A normally active person might have been immobilized by a pelvic fracture, for example, which led to a pneumonia and subsequent demise. Is that considered a death by pneumonia or a death from accident?

What can or should be done to mitigate the statistics? Certainly, osteoporosis which thins and weakens the bones inviting fractures must be addressed and reversed. If active weight bearing exercises, like running, jogging, or walking, cannot be done adequately, measures must be taken to assure early diagnosis of osteoporosis so that corrective measures can be instituted. A bone density study is certainly a worthwhile test that can establish the diagnosis. Even without the test, all post-menopausal women should be on Vitamin D, calcium supplements, and a medication, like Fosamax, as usually prescribed by the family doctor or gynecologist. The Fosamax is being replaced by a stronger and better medication, called Denusomab (Prolia), which is administered as subcutaneous injection twice a year. Every post-menopausal woman should be on Prolia.

Senior men can also become osteoporotic if they are not doing weight bearing exercises and become seriously and inevitably osteoporotic if they need androgen deprivation therapy to treat prostate cancer. Denusomab injections must become part of their regime.

Canadians may not get enough vitamin D from sunshine and may thus be vulnerable to rickets. Global warming may change this but, in the meantime, supplemental calcium, vitamin D and Denosumab make sense for all senior men who are not getting enough weight bearing exercise and sunshine. If they are on androgen deprivation therapy because of prostate cancer, Denosumab becomes mandatory.

Accidents that can be fatal are very often due to the automobile. The movement towards driverless cars should help as should the sophisticated technology built into the latest vehicles that lessen the chances of vehicles crashing into anything. But, while advances continue to occur in technology to reduce the chances of a fatal accident, impaired driving under the influence of alcohol, marijuana, or insufficient sleep continue to bewitch the driving public.

It seems to me reasonable to have a breath analyzer apparatus for private use by the driver in addition to that by a police officer. Would a driver continue to drive if he knew he had a high blood alcohol reading? Perhaps a device to detect degree of dexterity can also become part of self- assessment. Would anyone continue to drive knowing he is impaired? As we move more and more into the era of the driverless cars with its reduced risks of fatal accidents, there are more and more reports of the deliberate use of automobiles as battering rams to maim and kill innocent bystanders, by deranged people or terrorists. Are we actually evolving as a species? Could that be a myth?

Bottom line: It is fortunate that, to date, war, natural disasters, and famine have not made it to the list of the ten most common causes of deaths in Canada. Still, with the reality of global warming finally sinking in it is only a question of time before man made weather issues will impact mankind. When will we awaken to the realization that in order to survive as a species, petty quarrels based on misplaced loyalties must cease?

Over the years, young men of almost every country and nationality have been cajoled into believing he must sacrifice his life to fulfil the political objectives of his political leaders. Young Americans who refused to go to war in Viet Nam were the exceptions. Some of them ended up in Canada and, I think, made our country better. Cassius Clay or Mohammed Ali, the boxer, said: "I have no quarrels with the Viet Cons." How prescient! We need more people who will challenge the wisdom of political leaders, the wisdom of military might, the taking of innocent human lives! Donald Trump often refers to the Corona virus, Covid-19, as the China virus: should we then not call all nuclear bombs the American bomb?

Six: Diabetes

I am not surprised to see Diabetes listed as one of the ten most common causes of death in Canada. It is number six. The disease is very common as one form, the type 2 diabetes, is related to excess body weight, an epidemic problem of our civilization. Type 1 diabetes is an inherited disease manifesting first in childhood. In this disorder, insulin, a hormone normally made by certain cells in the pancreas cannot be made or processed properly leading to high levels of sugar in the blood normally kept at an acceptable level by insulin. The disease has many manifestations as might be expected in a population whose vasculature is, in fact, twenty percent older than their chronological age. (That is the one and only statement I remember from a medical school lecture on the subject.) Thus, heart attacks, strokes, kidney diseases, vision problems, blocked circulation, and skin disorders are all common consequences of the disease.

It may be appropriate here to mention the metabolic syndrome, an epidemic disorder of our times in the western world. The syndrome is characterized by a combination of the following: excess weight from too much fat, particularly about the waist, elevated blood pressure, high cholesterol levels in the blood, and an increased tendency to develop certain illnesses, like prostate cancer, diabetes, and dementia.

Type 2 diabetes can be prevented by appropriate weight reduction and vigorous exercise. The appropriate diet should be rich in whole grain and fiber, high in polyunsaturated fats found in nuts, vegetable oils, and fish. There should be restriction of sugary beverages, red meat and other sources of saturated fat. Smoking should cease. The goal of the exercise is to get the Hemoglobin A1C level to 6.5% or lower.

Measurement of hemoglobin A1C has largely replaced measurement of blood glucose levels in recent times. There must be a good reason for this change but I don't know what it is. Hemoglobin A1C readings reflect the average blood glucose level of the past three months. The results are rendered in percentage. Readings under 5.7% are considered normal. When the results are over 6%, that person is considered pre-diabetic and when the results are over 6.5%, the candidate is diabetic. A wearable device not unlike a wristwatch can make A1C readings when it is held over the skin, not even touching it. The device must be very welcome to those who hated the needle punctures.

Every adult Canadian knows about Frederick Banting and the story of how he introduced insulin to treat diabetes. He was awarded a Nobel prize in Medicine, an award he had to share with McLeod. And, therein, lies an oft repeated tale of work and reward. By the time Banting became involved with this potentially lethal medical problem it was known that the pancreas produced a product that controlled the level of blood sugar. It was already named and called insulin. Attempts to extract insulin from the pancreas where it was known to be produced were, at first, unsuccessful because the digestive enzymes produced by the pancreas destroyed the sugar controlling chemical which is insulin. One scientist tied off the duct in the pancreas through which the enzymes flowed and was able to extract the sugar controlling product.

Banting and Best, (his young assistant) succeeded in producing sufficient amount of insulin employing this technique for a successful human trial. Banting was awarded the Nobel prize and he shared his prize money with Best, but was bitter that McLeod, in whose laboratory the work was done, was equally rewarded. McLeod split his Nobel prize money with Collip, the biochemist who was helpful in the venture because it was in Collip's lab that the sugar was measured. The proper allocation of rewards and honors following a scientific advance is always a difficult task. Why didn't the person who first suggested tying off the pancreatic duct, for example, get more recognition?

No question, the introduction of insulin in clinical practice was revolutionary and Banting deserves much credit. He could have been more Canadian about it, though. (In another section I will discuss Wilhelm Kolff and the invention of the artificial kidney. Kolff deserved more credit than he got, in my view.)

The medications used today to treat type 1 diabetes is insulin and for type 2 diabetes, Metformin. Insulin is no longer produced by extraction from other animals. It is manufactured by bacteria bio-engineered to produce a specific chemical product. Metformin decreases the production of glucose by the liver, increases oxygen released into a cell, and increases the body's sensitivity to insulin. In type 2 diabetes, metformin is prescribed usually with one of the long acting insulin.

In recent times, it has been recognized that Metformin may also be an anti-aging agent as well. One 500 mg pill taken twice a day may actually contribute towards longevity. Studies are underway right now to make that determination. The chances of a positive result, that is, longer lives, with metformin seems very likely. After all, diabetic patients on Metformin were determined to live longer than people, otherwise matched, who were not diabetic and therefore, not taking Metformin. A larger study is underway with results expected in the very near future. It is likely to show that Metformin can lengthen life much more than competing preparations, such as Rapamycin, Reversatrol, or Acarbose, preparations also under study.

Despite better control of blood sugar levels, people's lives are frequently shortened by diabetes. This can be because of poor control of the sugar levels, or by injuries to the body vasculature. If we were serious about not having our lives shortened by diabetes, we just have to make certain we better control our body weight. We can't do much about childhood diabetes, but adult diabetes is a totally controllable disease, but it requires more dedicated mental discipline than most adults can supply.

So, what can be done to ascertain that our lives will not be shortened by diabetes? Choose appropriate parents to avoid childhood diabetes for one. That is a facetious answer. The reality is that we are not too far from being able to manipulate genetic inheritance. To apply the science to childhood diabetes makes more sense to me than to apply it to choose the sex of an offspring. As far as adult diabetes is concerned, the science has been solved. Implementing the science requires mental discipline not yet within our full control. That will come or should come. It is a curious fact that most people are interested in lengthening their lifespan, but simple maneuvers, like reducing unnecessary food intake becomes an impossible challenge for them.

Bottom line: The genetics of childhood diabetes is well understood: it seems to me likely that gene manipulation can and will solve the problem. If I were a potential parent and had a choice whether to pass on juvenile diabetes to the next generation, I would welcome an opportunity not to do so. I know that not everybody will agree with me. Adult diabetes is akin to a weight problem and we know that not everybody will have the mental discipline to conquer the problem. Insulin and Metformin, though, have transformed the lives of many diabetics.

Metformin is emerging as a life-lengthening product with no negative consequences, as far as I know. With experts in the field, like David Sinclair, on it, I have decided to take it myself. I am convinced there can be no negative consequences. It is also generic and inexpensive. The worst that can happen, in my opinion, is that it may prove ineffective. Other competing products, though, are not worth their high costs in my estimation.

Death from adult diabetes could and should be transformed by better adult weight control. Who is at fault when we lack this control? Is it the individual who should know better? Is it the world of commerce that prioritize profit over health? Is it the individual citizen or is it poor leadership? It is interesting to speculate on these questions: perhaps as important as determining whether the Corona virus, Covid-19, came from bats or rats.

Lifespan shortened by adult diabetes makes no sense to me. To me, it is like declining vaccination when smallpox is rampant! I don't know why the vasculature in diabetics is twenty percent older than their actual age. That is a fact, though, and that is why diabetics are more likely to have to undergo an amputation of a limb, or a cardiac revascularization. If you do not want your life shortened by adult diabetes, get rid of the excess weight.

Seven: Alzheimer's Disease

Alzheimer's disease is listed as the 7th most common cause of death in Canada. It is certainly the most common cause of dementia. One out of every four person,

male or female, over the age of 80 will develop Alzheimer's disease. The disease occurs slightly more often in women compared to men. This has been linked to the loss of estrogen after menopause although the connection is not that strong. Nevertheless, I foresee the return of hormone replacement therapy in women as the risk of breast cancer is not nearly as worrisome as once believed and the benefits of estrogen (less bladder infection, better sex life, and now, less Alzheimer) are substantial, in my view.

The afflicted victim of Alzheimer's disease will have short term memory issues, difficulty performing simple tasks, and exhibit bizarre behavior. The deterioration is progressive, but the speed of progression will be quite variable. There are people who have struggled with this disease for over a decade and others who were gone in a matter of months. We know what the brain of the Alzheimer victim looks like, it is shriveled with scattered deposits of amyloid, or amyloid-like products, but we don't know what causes the disease nor ways to reverse or prevent the changes.

A few medications, like Aricept tablets and Exelon patches have been developed, but their effectiveness are at most, marginal. The afflicted victim becomes an enormous burden to the other family members who must tend to their basic needs even as they become a stranger to the disease victim. We are in dire, desperate need for a scientific break-through for this nasty affliction. At present, all we have is a list of what are considered healthy food for the brain (green leafy vegetables, nuts, beans, berries, whole grain, fish, poultry, olive oil, and wine), and unhealthy foods for the brain (red meat, butter, cheese, pastries and sweets, fried fast foods). How much we actually gain by paying attention to this nutritional information is unclear, although the list seems to me to be no different from what might be advised to maintain a healthy heart.

We need a break-through in our understanding and treatment of Alzheimer's disease. One in four when over eighty is just too high a prevalence. Unless there is a break-through, the statistics are going to worsen as the population ages, more and more. Recently there was a report that a medication made by the pharmaceutical firm, Biogen, may help victims of Alzheimer's disease. The initial results of this preparation were not positive and the product was supposed to have been abandoned. However, it appears that the trial continued and the most recent studies showed positive results. We can only hope that it is for real.

As we age, it is normal to become more forgetful. Where are those damn keys? But, that is not Alzheimer's! The forgetfulness in Alzheimer's more bizarre as is the behavior. "What is your name?" you might be asked, moments after talking about it. And why is there so much struggle to put on a hat, he or she is not going anywhere! Alzheimer's disease is the most dehumanizing disease I can think of. The victim behaves like a child flailing against a loving parent. The mental deterioration can afflict any victim regardless of education or previous accomplishments. The victim can turn against the very family members who are struggling to help him or her. And, for now, there is no worthwhile treatment.

Bottom line: as I have already indicated I fear Alzheimer's more than I do any other malady. Should I develop it and cannot recognize family members I would want my life terminated. My attitude may change with newer medications, though. We can always hope.

Eight: Influenza and Pneumonia

INFLUENZA

How much does the average doctor know about influenza? Probably a lot less than a curious citizen who has checked the internet. As Medical students we learned that influenza is due to a virus, which are tiny pathogenic organisms significantly smaller than a bacteria. A virus cannot be seen under a regular microscope whereas a bacteria can be stained and seen. Furthermore, bacteria can live inside or outside a cell, unlike a virus that can live only inside live cells. The influenza virus changes slightly from year to year, and three types that affect mankind are recognized, called type A, type B, and type C. Yearly outbreaks of influenza affect 3 to 5 million people around the world and kill about 250.000 to 500,000 people.

Larger outbreaks occur from time to time and are called pandemics. The memorable ones are the Spanish flu of 1918 associated with 50 million deaths, the Asian influenza of 1957 with 2 million deaths, and the Hong Kong influenza in 1968 with 1 million deaths. We don't know yet how many victims Clovid-19, the Corona virus will claim particularly because we don't yet have any valid therapeutic options. We do know that these viruses are spread through the air when an affected person coughs or sneezes into another person's mouth, nose, or eyes. The virus can also be spread by touching contaminated surfaces, like tabletops or doorknobs, and bringing the hand to the eyes or mouth. This mode of virus transmission has been determined to be far less common than that due to normal respiration or coughing. Thus, facial masks and social distancing may be the most significant behavioral change necessary to limit the contagion, while coughing into the elbow and frequent hand washings have become part of normal living.

In the case of the influenza virus, after an incubation period of about 2 days the affected victim will develop a cough, chills, body aches, and fever. Sometimes, it is difficult to distinguish a flu from a cold. Usually, though, a cold does not cause muscle aches or fever. The distinction can be difficult because one third of people with influenza can be symptom-free. Viral shedding peaks on day two and symptoms peak on day three.

Tamiflu (oseltamir), taken early can abort or lessen the severity of the illness. Amantadine, available since 1966, is recognized as an effective anti-viral drug, and a few other drugs are available, but the majority of victims do well with just rest, hydration, and Tylenol or Aspirin. Remember that the virus can survive for a time on different surfaces but can replicate only within living cells.

Recently, a new virus has emerged out of China. It is a Coronavirus and has been named COVID-19. It has already become a frightening world-wide pandemic with fatalities increasing daily. Almost every part of the civilized world is reporting cases which is spread much the way influenza is spread. Washing ones hands a minimum twenty seconds with soap and water, wiping contaminated surfaces with alcohol swabs, and surgical masks are all mandatory to limit the spread. Social spacing, keeping two yards away from any human contact, is a concept very foreign to our civilization. The lethal nature of this new virus, though, has frightened the world into responsible behavior. Whether the virus will be contained or whether its spread will cause countess deaths remains to be determined. I can't remember the last time potentially exposed people were isolated into hastily contrived quarters for several weeks. These measures are imposed on people returning from countries with known problems, like China and Iran. Will the measures contain the contagion? We do not yet know how many lives will be taken by this alarming virus, but the contagion already qualifies as a pandemic. A vaccine will be developed for certain, but how many victims the virus will claim before it is contained by vaccination or by newly developed drugs? A worthwhile vaccine is still a year or a year and half away (2021?) according to the experts. Our faith in a successful vaccine may also be over-rated. Annual vaccination against the flu, after all, is not uniformly successful.

I hope an effective vaccine will be developed against the Corona, Clovid-19, virus. The pandemic it has caused has already taken half a million lives (June 2020). Scientists and politicians from around the world have come together to make certain we won't have a disaster like that caused by the Spanish flu of 1918. Is success likely? I think so. As a species mankind has conquered micro-organisms far better than he has resolved political squabbles.

The pandemic caused by Clovid-19, the Corona virus, has challenged humanity to change its behavior once again. Can we, as a species, keep our distance from one another, can we postpone planned trips indefinitely, can we wash our hands repeatedly with soap and water for twenty seconds, can we keep our hands away from our faces, learn to cough into our elbows, and can we keep doing all that for weeks, if not for months?

There is so much we do not yet know about the Corona virus. Will we be able to develop an effective vaccine? Will there be an effective anti-viral treatment? Is Clovid-19 going to take under a million lives, or will it be like the Spanish flu that killed 50 million people! How much warning do we need, as a species, to get our act together? Why can we not have a movement promoting humanity at all cost! It could start with the elimination of all stockpiles of nuclear arsenal!. Our very survival as a species will depend upon our responses to the threat of global warming, attacks from micro-organisms, and the flourishing of personal greed. Will we, as a species, be up to the challenge?

PNEUMONIA

So, you might ask, what can I tell you about pneumonia that you don't already know (or what will not be totally boring to you). You already know that pneumonia can be due to bacteria, viruses, or fungi that settle in the breathing sacs within the lung and which are called alveoli. With pneumonia alveoli fill with fluid or pus. The afflicted person may have chest pain, cough, fatigue, shortness of breath, nausea, vomiting, and fever. Anybody can get pneumonia but the most vulnerable population are children under two and seniors over seventy. Also vulnerable are those whose immune system is compromised, like people fighting AIDS or organ rejection after an organ transplantation. Immunization against bacterial and viral pneumonia are available but there is no immunization against pneumonia due to a fungus.

Pneumonia is often further defined by a prefix. Thus, bronchopneumonia defines a disease that affects mainly the bronchi, the tubing that leads to the alveolus. Aspiration pneumonia means food meant for the digestive tract ended up in the breathing tube where it does not belong, causing serious, life-threatening trouble. Hospital acquired pneumonia means that the offending bacteria are resistant to all the regular antibiotics available.

The distinction between pneumonia and influenza is, at times, difficult. Influenza is more likely to be seasonal and more widespread within a community. Pneumonia can more often claim lives because they are often problems in people fighting other health issues, like cancer, stroke, or major organ failure. It is often the terminal event. The diagnosis can usually be made by the treating physician, but a chest x-ray, CT scan, or bronchoscopy may be necessary, at times, to further clarify the situation. It would not be unreasonable if a sputum culture was ordered or measurement of oxygen saturation by sensors on fingertips.

What can we do to lessen the chances of having our own lives shortened by influenza or pneumonia? Immunization, when possible, is always worthwhile. Should influenza or pneumonia occur, aggressive treatment should be instituted as soon as possible. Every attempt must be made to avoid complications, like sepsis (high temperature), lung abscess, pleural effusion, and respiratory failure that can lead to kidney failure and/or heart failure. Supportive measures to lessen the burden, like ventilators and oxygen tanks, also make sense. Precautionary measures, like coughing into a napkin, frequent hand-washings, antiseptic (alcohol) cleansing of contaminated tabletops, phones, and doorknobs all make sense and should be routine and universal.

Bottom line: Influenza or pneumonia can be a life threatening disorder particularly in someone fighting a serious disease. It is often an associated terminal event. What can any individual do to lessen his chances of becoming a victim of pneumonia and influenza? Whenever possible, get immunized. Immunization may never be one hundred percent effective but it is virtually one hundred percent safe

Nine: Suicide

Suicide is the ninth most common cause of death in Canada. That statistic must include the Inuit population whose suicide rate is astronomical! It is a national disgrace that the suicide rate should be so high in the Inuit community especially as those taking their lives are so often young teen-agers. How can fellow Canadians feel comfortable isolating them in communities without running water and electricity? I know that allocation of federal funds meant to improve their condition often do not reach the proper destination, but that certainly must be a correctable problem or must be made a correctable problem. There is a widely held perception that government funds meant for the aboriginal population, like the North American Indians as well as the Inuits, do not always reach the proper destination. Is that a fact? Can we not determine the facts. If their leaders or people in their community are lining their own pockets, we should know that too. If that is an incorrect accusation, we should know that as well. We need to know the truth.

In my lifetime I have seen more and more Inuit and North American Indian personalities being interviewed on radio and television. It is obvious from their remarks that they are no different from other citizens that make up the country. So, why should they be treated differently? Why do they live in remote settlements with no running water? Why should they be paying less for alcohol and cigarette – isn't that an encouragement to drink and smoke more? Why don't aboriginal rights extend to making them more like any other citizen?

There are statistics about suicides that are totally baffling to me. Why do men commit suicide three times more often than women? Why is the suicide rate for men highest when they are in their forties, and then, after they are ninety? Why is suicide rate for women highest when they are in their fifties? Why is the rate of suicide higher in Russia than anywhere else in the world, higher even than in our Inuit population?

Suicide is totally bizarre to me; I don't understand it, never have understood it, and it continues to baffle me. Life is such a precious blessing why would anybody want to end it prematurely? I can recall every case of suicide I have encountered in my lifetime: I cannot say that about other deaths. I don't remember all the cases of "drownings" of people I have known, for example, or of those who have died in motor vehicle accidents, or airplane crashes, or even heart attacks. But, every single case of suicide among people I have known is memorable to me for different reasons, and every one of them was carried out by seemingly normal rational people. Let me go over them.

In 1942, every Canadian of Japanese ancestry living on the west coast of Canada was interred in interior British Columbia, at least one hundred miles from the coast so that they could not commit sabotage, aiding the Japanese military, the argument went. About one thousand of the twenty-two thousand Japanese-Canadians thus displaced ended up in Quebec - like our family. Two Japanese-Canadian men, then in their late sixties or, perhaps, seventies hanged themselves from the ceiling of their apartment in Montreal in 1947. What led them to take this action remains a mystery. I don't know if the first encouraged the second, or if there was any connection between the two suicides. What was it that made their situation unbearable when it was not unbearable during their period of incarceration?

Two young men committed suicide the year after graduating from the medical school at Queen's University in Kingston, Ontario. I knew them both rather well, better than I knew many of their fellow classmates. The year was 1963 and I was in Kingston doing a senior year of training in Urology. I needed an apartment as I was about to be married and the hospital quarters were no longer suitable. The very first senior medical student I met in Kingston introduced me to an available duplex just above his. It was furnished and owned by an absentee landlord, and we were fortunate to get it. The student was married and had a charming, attractive wife and a baby daughter. He interned somewhere in Ontario, I am not certain where, and he took his life during the year of his internship. I am unaware of any further details. A second student from the same class ended up interning in Montreal at the hospital I called "home." He was a bright and conscientious student, obsessed about tidiness. He also had a habit of scratching his head, in one particular area, to the point of creating a bald spot. During the year of his internship, he carefully sealed a room in his apartment, pumped exhaust from his car into the room and ended his life. I am mystified what persuaded him to do this at that particular time in his life. I believe he already had a position to train in Ophthalmology at McGill.

I have known three established doctors who committed suicide in Montreal. One was a urologist-radiologist, a colleague, and friend. He was found with his wife inside his car in a closed garage with the engine running. Rumour had it that his wife had recently developed dementia. Was that the reason for the presumed double suicide? I don't know and I am unaware whether any notes were left. A family doctor I knew who practiced just outside the city of Montreal (and sent me many referrals) jumped off the roof of his apartment building. There was no obvious explanation for his action. Rumour had it that he took a licking in the stock market. In like fashion, a skilled cardiovascular surgeon, who left Montreal for the USA, jumped to his death. There was no obvious reason for his suicide as well. Rumor had it that like all new arrivals, he was referred the horrible cases established surgeons shunned. How many doctors have killed themselves because they thought they could have served their patients better?

Two brothers from a good family in Montreal both deliberately drowned themselves a few years apart. The father never recovered from these events, but the mother became a counsellor to help others in similar circumstances.

I have been asked a number of times if I could help expedite the demise of a patient because he or she had an advanced illness, was in severe pain and distress, and there was no further worthwhile therapeutic option. I have prescribed high doses of narcotics on these occasions more than likely hastening their demise. I do not understand the current controversy regarding assisted suicides. Accepting and understanding the Hippocratic Oath should be sufficient for any doctor, in my view, to deal with the problem. Do not all doctors take the oath to serve our patients to the best of our ability and does that not include medications that might hasten the demise of a suffering patient?

Let me relate the most bizarre case of suicide I have encountered. The subject was a gentleman patient and a friend! He lived nearby and he knew where I lived. On one of his visits to my office he said he had noticed cracks in my cement walkway. "You better fix those cracks before you have a foundation problem in your house ," he warned me. I thanked him but did nothing to repair the cracks. One day he arrived in his fancy car, and personally fixed the cracks with tools and cement he had brought with him. On another visit to the office he said I need not worry about him. "What do you mean?" I asked. "I have put away enough sleeping pills to end my life when the time comes," he said. A short time later he took his wife to a luxury hotel just outside the city and smothered her to death with a pillow. He was certain she had Alzheimer's disease. There was a trial and he was incarcerated. Upon his release he went to his wife's grave site, poured gasoline on himself and lit the match. He never used the pills he said he had accumulated and chose a much more painful way to go... as if he needed to punish himself.

Life is a precious commodity. Why would anyone deliberately abandon it? Consider what is required to raise a newborn child anywhere in the world. Babies have to be fed, changed, cuddled and comforted just to make it to the next day. I have long felt that hardened criminals should be made to care for infant children. Not one child can survive without helping hands. Perhaps anyone who still feels that his life must end and cannot be persuaded otherwise, despite extensive professional counsel, should be allowed to become an organ donor. Let his heart, lungs, kidneys, pancreas, lens, skin, bone marrow, blood and whatever else support the life of those of us who will carry on.

As a Canadian of Japanese origin, I am particularly aware that the Japanese military championed suicides, encouraging young men to volunteer for the "Kami-kaze" (godly winds) missions that antedates current suicide attacks by Islamic extremists. Is it not interesting that these missions were never carried out by men passed middle age as far as I know. Older men, even elderly men are capable of carrying out suicide missions. Why does that not happen? Could it be that by middle age most people acquire enough common sense to question the wisdom of such an inhumane action?

As our population ages, one of the inevitable health problems we confront is dementia, which, along with heart disease, cancer, and diabetes becomes epidemic. But, with dementia, we lose our ability to participate in decisions regarding artificial prolongation of life. Do people who can no longer recognize their own spouse or children want to carry on living indefinitely? Isn't it interesting that people with severe dementia can still remember how to chew food, how to walk, how to move their bowels and bladder? What is the definition of a sentient being? When should the challenge to prolong life cease, if ever?

I am willing to have extraordinary measures tried to restore my health should I develop a serious illness, like a cancer, but I do not wish such measures implemented in the face of severe dementia. If I can no longer recognize family, expedite my departure. Use the resources to help others.

Did you think I had more suicide tales to tell? I do not. Violent deaths from firearms, though, is worthy of further comment. Why are Americans so fixated on the right to bear arms to the point they have lost all common sense in the eyes of the rest of the world. I have never owned a gun and have no desire to own one. I fired a pistol once in my life, as a medical cadet in training. The year was 1956. I got no thrill from it and it is unlikely I will do it again in my lifetime. Why should the right to bear arms extend to semi-automatic, military killing machines? What is wrong with a society that cannot distinguish hunting rifles from machine-guns? Why are Americans so intimidated by the NRA (National Rifle Association)? Will the student movement finally curb their control of American life? (Earlier in my life I had a number of offers to move to a more lucrative, possibly more prestigious practice in the USA. I am not sorry I never did.)

Do I have any suggestion on how we might reduce our incidence of suicides? I do not. From the stories I have heard, though, it would appear that many people who have tried but failed to end their lives end up with a renewed interest in life, pleased, in fact, that their attempt had failed. Thus, access to professional help is what needs to be always available and accessible.

We can learn from communities with established records of good health and longevity. They interacted and socialized abundantly with their neighbours. Are our children and grandchildren who interact more with their cell phones than with "real" people at increased risk for suicides? I sure hope not.

Bottom line: people of any age contemplating suicide must have immediate access to professional counselling. Those who have attempted suicide and failed often live with a renewed interest in life. What should be done about our native population whose suicide rates, especially among young women, is unacceptably sky high? Is professional counselling all that we need to correct the problem? I suspect something more dire is at play. I earnestly hope the problem will be addressed and corrected.

Suicides and fatal accidents are outcomes we should be able to change as sentient beings. Suicides, after all, are extraordinary brave acts in a moment of folly while fatal accidents are so often an astonishingly foolish act, in a fragmentary moment of time. As a rule neither would have occurred with more deliberation. So, how could we have bought more time? The obvious answer: more social interaction! As our inanimate toys, like cell phones, become more and more animate, human beings, as a species, are becoming more and more inanimate, leery of one another, distrustful, paranoid, and unfriendly. We are, in fact, evolving a civilization more prone to suicides and fatal accidents. We must change that if we are to survive as a species.

There is an old line: "Any doctor who treats himself has a fool for a doctor." In like fashion: any suicide candidate who listens only to himself has a fool for an advisor: the perspective we give to our own problem is very often uneven and unwise. Seeking professional counsel is not a sign of weakness: it is a sign of intelligence.

Have I ever talked anybody out of committing suicide? Yes, I have and more than once, although I will never claim exclusive credit. "You must rethink this," I would argue, "we all make mistakes, that is what life is all about!"

Ten: Kidney Disease

Kidney disease is listed as the tenth most common cause of death in Canada. Was it number ten before the development of dialysis (artificial kidney) and kidney transplantation? I don't think so: it had to be much higher before. Wilhelm Kolff invented the artificial kidney in the early 1940's in the Netherlands. I have often wondered why this development occurred in the most war ravished country in Europe at the time. I am also puzzled why Kolff was never awarded the Nobel prize for his monumental achievement. I think it was certainly deserved. As crude as his original contraption might have been, it was the ingenious product of one man.

What exactly did Kolff do? He diverted blood from his uremic patient into a tubing made from sausage casings obtained from the local butcher shop. This tubing was wrapped around a wooden spool and the whole thing, tubing and spool, was immersed in an equivalent of a wash-tub filled with a solution that was like normal serum. When the uremic blood of his patient was passed through the tubing exchanges of chemicals took place so that the blood was lessened in its concentration of waste chemicals, like urea and creatinine. The sausage casing, in fact, functioned as a semi-permeable membrane, the essence of the artificial kidney.

How did Kolff come to think that he could normalize uremic blood? He was a young doctor just starting his practice when he had to look after a young woman in kidney failure. She probably had acute glomerulonephritis although I am not certain of that. He applied the treatment of the day which consisted of keeping such a patient in a darkened room, administered magnesium sulfate enemas to lower the very high blood pressure, watched the patient slip into a uremic coma and die. Just then, he attended a public lecture by a certain Dr. Brinkman, a physiologist. The topic of the lecture was semi-permeable membranes. When fluids of different composition are separated by a semi-permeable membrane, like cellophane (or sausage casings), the composition of the fluid on either side of the membrane will be altered because cells and large molecules cannot pass through the "pores" of the membrane but salts and small molecules will pass through the "pores" and equilibrate. In principle the process is not that different from when a tea bag is placed into a cup of hot water. The ingredients in the tea leaves that are responsible for the taste and color are passed into the hot water, but not the leaves themselves.

Kolff must have had an "Aha!" moment.

What if I took the blood of my uremic patient, placed it in a sac made of a semi-permeable membrane, and immersed the sac in a bath solution that mimicked normal serum, Kolff must have wondered. Will the uremic serum become normalized? Will chemical waste products, like creatinine and urea, that are normally eliminated by a healthy kidney but accumulate in the blood when the kidneys fail move into the bath water? He tried an experiment with a small sample of his patient's uremic blood. The blood sample of his patient was placed into a sausage casing sac and immersed into bath water that had the composition of normal serum. The uremic blood lost its heavy concentration of waste chemicals. Indeed, the abnormal blood became more normal – the urea and the creatinine level in the serum dropped dramatically. The uremic blood was becoming more normal. He then set out to build an "artificial kidney" to do what he had accomplished - on a larger scale!

He obtained sausage casings from the local butcher shop, wrapped the tubing around a wooden drum and immersed the drum with its tubing into a tub filled with a solution that simulated normal blood serum. The waste chemicals, like creatinine, urea, and uric acid moved into the bath water while the blood within the casing normalized. The "artificial kidney" was born.

There is an interesting Montreal aside to this story. When Kolff built a few extra "artificial kidneys" to be tried out elsewhere, one was sent to the Royal Victoria Hospital (my hospital) in Montreal. How that came about was as follows. Dr. Gavin Miller was the chief of Surgery at the Royal Victoria at that time. He was a larger-than-life figure, often doing several operations at the same time, running from one theatre to another making the critical maneuvers. When he heard about Kolff's invention, he wrote to him. I have seen the original letter but, unfortunately, it has since been lost.

I do remember the gist of its content, though. Miller wrote that Montreal had its share of patients with kidney failure. Montreal was a city of over one million people, half English-speaking and half, French-speaking, he wrote. If you were to send your "invention" here, we will be pleased to try it out. Kolff wrote back that he will send his "artificial kidney" if the hospital was also willing to accept a lady doctor who wanted to emigrate to Canada. The deal was made, and the crude contraption did come to the hospital as did the doctor.

Kolff's kidney launched a search for other semi-permeable or dialyzing membranes that might be tried. One possibility was the inner lining of the small intestine, called the intestinal villi. American investigators had disconnected half the length of the small intestine. A person's digestive needs could be fulfilled by a small intestine shortened by fifty percent. The two ends of the disconnected portion of the small intestine were brought out to the skin as a stoma (like patients with excised bowel and consequent ileostomy or colostomy). A solution like that used in the artificial kidney was dripped in the top opening and allowed to collect at the other end. During the transit it was hoped that the uremic waste might be lessened. It worked but not for long! The intestinal villi morphed into venous lakes and stopped behaving like a dialyzing membrane after about one week. Science was at this point when I proposed we try using the entire length of the small intestine by constructing two Roux-Y joints at the upper and lower end of the entire small intestine.

A Roux-Y anastomosis means that the bowel is interrupted, the opened distal end is brought to the skin to form a stoma, and the amputated proximal end is rejoined perhaps six inches or so beyond the skin opening distally. This meant that the bowel was shortened by a few inches, but ingested food will make its normal transit through the system and not pour out the opening because of the one-way traffic in the gut known as peristalsis. When this construction was carried out at the upper and lower end of the small intestine, it allowed fluid to be dripped in at the upper opening and collected at the lower opening. Perhaps, I thought, if the bowel processed food when it was not cleansing the blood, it may work better and longer as a dialyzing membrane.

The procedure had some success and was tried in several health centers in different cities in Canada and became known as the "Taguchi loop." I earned considerable notoriety as I was a junior resident at the time.

It turned out that a far better dialyzing membrane was the peritoneal lining within the abdomen although the risk of peritonitis was a real and constant threat. Peritoneal dialysis is still a therapeutic option when the kidneys fail. Dialyzing fluid is instilled into the abdomen, allowed to sit for a while, and then drained out. Daily or nightly peritoneal dialysis competes with thrice weekly hemodialysis to maintain kidney function when the kidneys fail.

Kidney transplantation, though, was an even better solution for the problem. With three relatively simple connections, that of the artery, vein, and ureter, a donor kidney can be placed in the lower abdomen to lie almost besides the bladder.

I have had a long connection with kidney transplantation, earning a doctorate in transplantation biology after demonstrating that overwhelming the recipient with donor specific protein can abort the rejection process in a rat kidney transplantation model. I was not able to get similar results with a dog model and abandoned the project. Still, I developed a simple way to connect the ureter to the bladder in the rat and tried it out, successfully, in a human recipient. I then reported it. Around the world this simple technique is commonly used to-day when Argentinian doctors reported that the technique was simpler to carry out and produced better results than other established techniques. It is known to-day as the "**Taguchi U-stitch.**"

The kidney remains the organ most frequently transplanted as just three connections are necessary, that of the artery, vein, and ureter. When the donor kidney is not from an identical twin, immunosuppressive drugs are necessary to suppress the rejection process. It was the drug called Imuran that launched organ transplantation from a donor who was not an identical twin. Over the years, more and better drugs have been developed and organs besides the kidney have been successfully transplanted from donors to recipients. The Royal Victoria Hospital, in Montreal, had, at one time, the second largest cadaver source kidney transplant series in the world. We were second only to Denver Colorado in the USA that did more. (I might also mention here that the Royal Victoria Hospital in Montreal was also the first hospital in the British Commonwealth to carry out a kidney transplantation from one identical twin to another. Joe Luke was the vascular surgeon and Ken MacKinnon the urologist when this took place in 1959.)

Cadaver kidneys were scarce and we made ourselves available to harvest them no matter when or where. The cardiologist would declare the arrest of the heartbeat, and that would signal us (the organ procurers) to rush the body to the operating room where we would paint and drape the body as if for an operation and try to retrieve the kidneys with their vessels and ureter intact as quickly as we possibly could.

Sometimes later, brain death became the criterion to qualify a body to be an organ donor as long as there was documented consent from the donor or consent from the immediate family. Removing kidneys from a brain dead donor, though, was not the same as removing organs from a body after a cardiac arrest. The body of a brain dead donor appeared to "object" to the surgical assault. The heart rate would speed up and the blood flow in the artery would become more bounding - as if in protest! There may even be a reflex jerk of a body or leg muscle. Did we really have consent for the mutilating procedure? I did not enjoy harvesting kidneys from brain-dead donors. Fortunately, for me, organ harvesting is a young man's game and I was getting a little too "senior" for it.

There is renewed debate on what constitutes brain death. Some countries, like Japan, does not allow an apparent brain death to define the demise of an individual. The lack of brain stem activity is sufficient for most countries, but it is hard to accept the finality of "death" in a youth on a ventilator with rosy cheeks.

Dialysis three times a week or a kidney transplant can replace kidney
function. Thus any disease that eliminates kidney function does not translate into an inevitable demise as was the case before these two developments. Diseases that can destroy kidney function are still not uncommon, though. They include glomerulonephritis, polycystic kidney disease, and severe hydronephrosis. In glomerulonephritis, the body's immune response to a streptococcal bacterial infection targets the glomerulus, rather than the bacteria, destroying the filters. The glomerulus is the filter within the kidney, and there are about a million of them in each kidney.

Polycystic kidney disease is an inherited condition, passed on from one generation to the next by one dominant gene, meaning that any parent with the disease can pass it on to fifty percent of his or her children. In the disorder the kidneys grow cysts throughout the substance of the kidneys, and as the cysts enlarge, as they do, they compress and destroy normal kidney tissue. This is quite different from cortical cysts which occur on the surface of the kidney. This occurs in up to fifteen percent of the population at large and the cyst or cysts can grow to an enormous size, like that of a cantaloupe, at times, but they do not become cancerous, nor do they seriously damage kidney function. Occasionally, though, surface cysts are multiple, or have walls within them. These cysts can be cancerous and require surgery.

Hydronephrosis is a blow-up of the urine draining system at the level of the kidney because of a blockage to the normal flow. Years ago, the common cause was a neglected enlarged prostate gland. That is uncommon today and the most frequent cause of hydronephrosis is an incomplete blockage at the point where the sac draining the kidney, called the renal pelvis, meets the tube (ureter) which takes the urine from the kidney to the bladder.

This problem is usually unilateral so that even when it is severe enough to destroy one kidney the remaining one can supply all the function the body requires. A generous and compassionate donation of one kidney for transplantation does not impair overall kidney function. A severe infection of the kidneys, called pyelonephritis can damage kidney function but, more often, injures the kidneys without destroying them. Students are taught that infection in the absence of obstruction does not cause the kidneys to fail.

Kidney cancers occur in two forms. One form originates in the substance of the kidney cell and is called renal cell carcinoma. Early on, there are no symptoms and the diagnosis is made only by accident. As the cancer gets larger there may be pain in the flank or blood in the urine, or both pain and blood. The disease may be diagnosed by its spread lesions which occur, oddly enough, in the brain, lung, or bones, without totally destroying the kidney where it originated. The second malignancy of the kidney originates in the urinary lining and is called transitional cell carcinoma. It is like a tumor of the bladder lining and can be just as lethal. As a rule, though, kidney cancers, whether it is a renal cell carcinoma or a transitional cell carcinoma are unilateral disease and become life threatening problems only if and when the disease becomes widespread.

Overall, cancers originating in the kidney, though not uncommon, are not common enough to warrant routine screening. At the same time, cancer is the first thing doctors think of when there is unexplained blood in the urine. Blood in the urine can be microscopic, that is, not visible to the naked eye. It can also be very obvious, especially if there are clots as well. Sometimes, a large serving of beets will cause the urine to look bloody but the color is a little different and the dip-stick urinalysis will indicate the absence of blood. Blood in the urine that cannot be seen by the naked eye is called microscopic hematuria. Sometimes, the condition is familial and not of concern. Persistent micro-hematuria requires investigation, in particular, a test called urine cytology. Three morning urine samples are collected and examined by trained experts for the presence of abnormal, that is, cancer cells.

Questionable results will lead to a cystoscopy, that is, an inspection of the interior of the bladder. A cystoscopy will also be necessary when the cytology is positive because there is a need to know how extensive and where the disease might be. Even people on blood thinners, with micro-hematuria, are advised investigation if their urine indicates the persistent presence of blood because a serious disorder will be found in ten to fifteen percent of cases.

So, are there measures that can be taken to lessen the

chances of having life shortened by kidney failure? Or, are such concerns unnecessary because of dialysis and transplantation? I think gene manipulation to eliminate polycystic disease of the kidney is going to become possible without sterilizing parents carrying the dominant gene. At least, I think and hope so. Some form of in-vitro fertilization may be necessary, but that is better than a one in two chance of passing it on. If I were a potential parent and had the opportunity of parenthood without passing on polycystic kidney disease, I would certainly embrace that possibility, and I suspect most parents would do so as well. Science has not yet found a way to prevent glomerulonephritis or Lupus, which can end in renal failure, but I think that can happen if enough resources were directed towards solving the problem. Perhaps some form of immunization will work. It is unfortunate that these health problems do not get the kind of research support cancer can get. Too bad!

A Note on Fetal Kidneys as Donor Organs

Earlier in my career I tried to explore the use of fetal kidneys as donor organs. There is an enormous shortage of donor organs to this day throughout the world. At the time, my hospital (the Royal Victoria) was the one carrying out mid-term abortions. I will not discuss here the pros and cons of pregnancy termination. That is another subject all together. Women from across the province were sent to the RVH for safe termination of their pregnancy. The aborted fetus was discarded in the hospital incinerator. I arranged to have the aborted fetus kept in cold saline.

I dissected out the kidney and transplanted the kidney into a laboratory rat. The fetal kidney had vessels and ureters the size of those in laboratory rats. It was a very difficult technical challenge but not an impossible one to carry out. Modification of the rejection process in a rat-to-rat kidney transplantation model was the subject of my PhD thesis. I then spoke to a number of patients in the Palliative Care ward of the hospital. I asked them if anyone might volunteer for an experiment that would involve freezing their arm, opening an area in the wrist (where the pulse is taken), installing a human fetal kidney which is about the size of a fingernail, and which may have to be removed in a second operation involving another freezing process. And all this will not contribute one iota to improve their own health. I was impressed with the willingness of many terminally ill patients to want to participate. But the hospital Ethics Committee heard of my intention and put a stop to it. As far as I know we are continuing to discard the aborted fetuses, and to this day I am not at all certain whether the transplant would have grown and worked. I do know that a fetal kidney at twenty weeks gestation produces urine which becomes part of the amniotic fluid.

Earlier, in 1963, we transplanted a kidney from a patient with liver failure into a recipient with kidney failure. There was nothing unusual about that except that before the transplantation, we had cross-circulated the blood of the two patients, that is, the blood flow from one arm of one patient was made to flow into the arm of the other patient and visa versa.

The weights of both patients were continuously monitored so that we tightened a clamp that reduced the flow in either direction if one patient was gaining weight. The kidney function in the renal failure patient improved and the liver failure patient was beginning to awaken from her hepatic coma. After about seventy-two hours of cross circulation the patient with the liver failure died rather suddenly, inexplicably. We transplanted one of her kidneys into the patient with the kidney failure as we had the consent to do so. The recipient never had a single rejection episode. I am certain this experiment would not be allowed today because of the stringent powers of the Ethics Committee. But, is that progress?

CHAPTER FOUR

Mistakes Are Lessons Learned

What are the mistakes I have made in my lifetime? There are plenty to be sure, some I am not yet ready to make public, but here are some I am willing to share. When I was in junior high school, I entered to run in a middle-distance race without a single practice run. There was only one other competitor. I took an early lead and heard the crowd cheer. Wow, I thought, maybe I can actually win this thing. At the mid-way point we were about even. My competitor passed me at the three-quarter mark and won the race by a country mile.

Lesson learned : No long distance race is determined by how you start the run!

In my lifetime, what is the most foolish decision I have ever made? I suspect it is this one which, earlier in life I would not have divulged because it was an admission of committing academic suicide!

I had the extraordinary honour of being the very first geographical full-time appointee in Urology at McGill. The year was 1966. A geographical full time appointment meant that you were assigned an office, a secretary, a salary, and you agreed to spend up to fifty percent of your time on academic activities, such as research and teaching, and not in clinical practice. I had a grant from the Medical Research Council of Canada and was working towards a doctorate in Investigative Medicine. I agreed to help run the kidney transplantation programme, continue my research, take on teaching assignments, and run an emerging clinical practice in Urology.

A few months later, a freshly trained general surgeon was appointed to run the kidney transplantation service with me. He already had a reputation for superb technical skills. He arranged to meet with me!

"I don't know anything about transplantation," he said. "You will have to teach me everything!"

"There's not much to it," I replied. "Besides, it's the medical guys who tinker with the medications. We just have to be ready to do the surgery and look after any complications."

In the course of our prolonged conversation that day, I found out that his salary was significantly more than mine. That did not make sense to me. I felt slighted and insulted. So, I took my complaint to my chief, the man I worshipped. I considered him my mentor – the man I regarded as the one who made me a urologist.

"I have no control of salaries," my chief said. "You must talk to the head of General Surgery." So, I did. But it turned out he didn't have any say either. He asked me to go talk to the dean. So, I did. But the dean said he had nothing to do with salaries and sent me back to the chief of Urology. So, I arranged another visit with my chief.

"I have no desire to leave Montreal, nor abandon Urology," I said, "but I no longer want to be involved in transplantation." My decision was accepted without rancour. In retrospect, the salary was a token recognition of my academic value. There was no recognized salary scale, my chief received no salary himself. The rules were in the process of being evolved.

It was an error for me to take the contract as a personal insult. As a Canadian of Japanese origin, though, I had already spent four years of my life in a detention camps in interior

British Columbia during World War II, and I was overly sensitive to unequal treatment based on racial origin. In reality, I would not be richer or poorer today because of the university salary and contract. I may have collected a university pension after retirement, but pensions are based on salaries, so it would not have amounted to much anyway.

In retrospect I made a foolish decision at the time. I had, in fact, committed academic suicide! At about this time in my life I was getting job offers from across the country. One head of Urology out west wanted me to join him with a promise that I would take over after his retirement which was imminent.

I turned down offers to work in Toronto, Vancouver, and Vermont, USA. The Vermont offer was interesting. I said you would be wasting your time trying to recruit me unless who can promise me exemption from military service. "We cannot promise that, but we can tell you that your chances of being drafted would be less than five percent." "Unless it's one hundred percent, you will be wasting your time," I said, and that was as close as I had ever gotten to moving to the USA.

Actually, that is not entirely correct. A few years later, I found out that my chief had been in talks with George Nagamatsu, a New York city academic urologist best known for developing a huge incision for removing kidney cancers. "I made a big mistake not getting you to come to New York," Dr. Nagamatsu said to me a few years later at a Urology meeting. Actually, my wife had spent some time as a nurse in New York city before moving to Montreal and I think she would have welcomed an opportunity to return to the big city.

Abandoning the geographical full-time appointment meant I relinquished not only the salary, but the office and the secretary. Still, I knew my craft well, I thought, and I could compete in the real world, which is all I ever wanted to do. I do wonder, at times, though, what kind of pension I would have drawn had I not abandoned my position in a huff. After all, the lesser salary offered to me was not because of ethnicity, accomplishments, or whatever else: it was simply not a serious consideration in a scheme that was in early development.

Summary – 10 Most Common Causes of Death in Canada:

So, there they are; the ten most common causes of death in Canada, what is commonly known about them, and what we can and cannot do about them . Besides these ten common causes of death, though, there may be other health problems that need to be discussed. Various attempts have been made to classify and stratify health disorders. One such classification is called SHIC, for Scale of Health and Illness Concerns. It recognizes ten levels of concern ranging from 0 for normal health to 10 for fatal illness. Here they are:

1. This level includes people with the metabolic syndrome, controlled stomach ulcer, Crohn's disease or ulcerative colitis, mild arthritis, controlled asthma, mild infirmities of age, like cataracts and partial hearing loss, and mild mental disorders, like attention deficit disorder.
2. Handicapped but managing, like someone virtually blind, or paraplegic.
3. Severe emphysema, COPD (chronic obstructive pulmonary disease), schizophrenia and depression controlled with medication.
4. Uncontrolled pain. Major problems with the gastro-intestinal, urinary, or respiratory tract.
5. Severe mental problems, like schizophrenia and depression that are uncontrolled despite treatment.
6. Serious cancer and cardiovascular disease

not controlled.

7. Established Alzheimer, Parkinson's, or other neuro-degenerative disease.

8. Quadriplegic or, for other reasons, continuously confined to bed.

9. Multiple organ failure, protracted coma, or incurable cancer.

10. Final stages of Alzheimer's, cancer, or AIDS.

It is not clear to me how a categorization like this clarifies serious health disorders in our country or help people wanting to live longer. It might have been better to list the twenty most common causes of death in Canada and to try to address problems inherent in causes 11 to 20. Such a list, though, does not appear to exist, at least, on the internet.

It is interesting to note that sexual dysfunction does not make the list. Certainly sexual problems are not life threatening issues but there is, undoubtedly a direct correlation of this problem with age. The dysfunction takes one of two forms: a lack of desire and/or a failure in performance. Lack of desire can affect either sex. It is often referred to as frigidity in the female and lack of libido in either sex. In both sexes the problem is commonly related to levels of testosterone in the body. Testing for testosterone levels can be troublesome. In my estimation the only valid reading would be the serum level of the bio-available testosterone taken in mid-morning, around ten to eleven AM. Should the reading be low (<30), testosterone administration as a skin patch, intramuscular injection, or intra-nasal squirt may fix the problem. The intra-nasal preparation, called Natesto is rapidly becoming to most popular preparation, although the intramuscular drug (Delatestryl) may be more economical.

Testosterone administration in men were traditionally frowned upon because of a fear of promoting prostate cancer. It has now been established that there is no risk of causing prostate cancer, but should prostate cancer be present, testosterone administration can cause the disease to spread.

Erectile dysfunction is the other aspect of the sexual problem. It is certainly a male issue. Over the years, before the introduction of Viagra (sildenofil) many ingenious tricks and dangerous devices were proposed, often by men suffering from the problem. As a urologist I encountered many of them. I have seen a glass stirring rod shoved into the urinary passage of the penis in an attempt to stiffen it, external stents strapped to the penis, blood sucked into the organ sustained by a tourniquet, etc. Injections of vasoactive drugs into the body of a flaccid penis was started by a senior urologist with the problem. It worked! A combination of one to three drugs could create a functional erection when injected into the body of the penis.

Patients were taught how to do the injection for themselves by a trained nurse, and almost every candidate succeeded. Also, an internal stent that could be hinged up and down or inflated by a pump installed in the scrotum were all procedures common to urologic practice. Most of these maneuvers were rendered obsolete with the introduction of Viagra.

I was taken to court once by an elderly gentleman who talked me into restoring his sex life by installing a penile prosthesis. Unfortunately, the procedure was complicated by a wound infection and the prosthesis had to be removed. In court, he declared that I had promised him a device that could be inflated and deflated by a press of a button. To this day I wonder if he believed he had such a conversation with me because it never occurred. The case was dismissed by the judge but it was, nevertheless, a trying and unpleasant experience for me.

CHAPTER FIVE

Doomsday

There is one other life- threatening health issue that I must mention here and this one is often man-made. They are problems that can move the arm of the dooms-day clock one notch closer to the critical midnight hour.

For some time now, perhaps a few decades and more, there have been forward-thinking people or doomsday preoccupied alarmists, depending on one's point of view, who have campaigned to prepare concerned citizens for the worst scenario: advising citizens to store bottled water, tinned sardines, and long lasting beeswax candles - the three ingredients essential to survive the first seventy-two hours when all utilities are rendered non-functional. Beyond that time period, what is necessary may be more controversial but, a manual tin-can opener, a hand-crank flashlight and battery radio, a water purification kit, gallons of stored petrol, a gasoline powered electricity generator, or one powered by the sun, a functional old fashioned automobile (ideally the kind you crank to start), an underground retreat, and finally, a "container" based dwelling in a remote country-side already prepared for such an eventuality. These are the things "experts" advise considering having on hand.

What are these disasters? A nuclear accident for one, an attack on the electricity grid up north for Canada is another, a mad-man with a miniature nuclear bomb in a suitcase (is that really possible?), an unanticipated, uncontrolled escalation of war-talk between quarreling nations ending up with the release of nuclear bombs, poisonous chemicals or virulent micro-organisms. When we consider the braggadocio of political leaders like Vladimir Putin, Donald Trump, and Kim Jong Un, the possibility of an accidental escalation does not seem so absurd or remote. Furthermore, the recent world-wide pandemic with the Corona virus (Covid-19) arising out of China with its many fatalities guarantees that global warming is not the only threat to mankind as we know it.

And, as far as natural disasters are concerned, there appears to be an increased frequency of earthquakes, volcanos, tornadoes, tsunami, floods and forest fires, as though planet earth is facing increasing difficulties coping with mankind's disrespect for mother-nature. Is that a fact or an erroneous perception of reality?

Does it make sense to spend time, money, and energy to prepare for such a disaster? Might we be better off to ignore such possibilities and concentrate our resources and energy instead on positive things we can do, like exercising more, eating better, helping our fellow citizens more, expanding our minds? I suppose time will tell which approach is or was the better one. Let us hope we can all live to talk about it.

In the meantime, might it not be prudent to spend a little time and effort on a minimum preparation. Storing bottled water (which I normally never use because I have no problems with tap water. My wife and children, though, insist on bottled water all the time), ascertaining a supply of long-lasting candles, and a supply of tinned sardines are things I have decided to do and to have on hand. A retreat in my back yard or the far north, though, is not something I am thinking of securing at this time although I am prepared to be persuaded to change my mind. We shall see and time will tell.

CHAPTER SIX

The Health Care Industry

L et us now examine the health care industry as it exists in Canada. Let me relate what I know of its structure, its strengths, its weaknesses, its triumphs, and its failures. This is a rather boring subject for most people, so I will interject anecdotes from my own life to try to keep your interest.

There is an abundance or, perhaps, too much tradition associated with the health care industry even in a relatively new country like Canada. I was a McGill medical student from 1955 to 1959 and I remember the welcoming address from the dean of the faculty at that time - Dr. Lyman Duff. He said each one of us was the successful one in seventeen or eighteen legitimate applicants that had applied. That was astounding as well as awesome! I also remember a lecture in my first or second year, I'm not certain which, when a classmate was dismissed from the lecture hall because he dared to attend without a jacket. I cannot imagine that happening today. Matted waist-long hair and jeans with holes, though, do not seem to me appropriate in a medical school classroom. Should there be a dress code then, or a uniform like those worn by private school attendees? I cannot imagine the students agreeing to it. In fact, if a student was dismissed from a classroom today because of a presumed dress code violation, there will be an uproar and the person most likely to be reprimanded would be the professor himself.

Anatomy, Histology, Physiology, and Biochemistry were the

subjects covered in the first year. All the professors dazzled us with their encyclopedic knowledge of their subject but that did not mean they all excelled in passing on their knowledge to the students. Often, the lectures were simply overwhelming and very definitely intimidating. Thinking about it now I am surprised the powers that be did not make the process of acquiring new knowledge more captivating, more interesting. Some did try, I must admit, and succeeded to some extent. But, it seems to me they were the exceptions - not the rule! Virtually all the students had, at a minimum, an undergraduate degree in one discipline or another. Those who had done an honors course in Physiology or Biochemistry were repeating the same course they had done before in their first year of med school. I don't know why the university was party to that. It wasn't good for them; they were repeating the course as if they had failed it the first time around. It wasn't good for those of us without that background: those few seemed to have extra advantages. They did not all necessarily continue to excel in later years, though.

I remember asking a question to the professor who taught us Histology, which is anatomy under the microscope. Curiously, I cannot remember what the question was. He smiled, I do remember, but pointedly declined to answer my question. I was baffled but did not pursue it further. The very question I had asked was on the exam a short time later. It's as though the professor did not want to give me any advantage and believed his behavior justifiable in a strange and peculiar way. Questions are better answered today on "Google" than by our teachers of that era.

The very same professor who declined to answer my question sought me out a short time later and asked me if I might want to work in his laboratory during the summer. I suspect it was because he liked my drawings. Unfortunately, I had to decline the offer because I had already joined the Canadian Air Force Reserve, as a medical cadet, simply because that assured me of a certain Summer job. I have often wondered what might have happened had I been able to accept his offer. The professor and the laboratory that made me the offer became world renowned at about that very time because it pioneered radio-isotope diagnostic tests. Would I have become an anatomist, a histologist, or some kind of lab man?

It is interesting how little events in life can shape a lifetime. I might not have become a Urologist, for example, had that not been my very first rotation in my first year of surgical training. If it had been left up to me I would not have picked Urology as my first rotation. I associated the specialty with foul smelling urine and bizarre instruments. I wanted to work with a scalpel! I did not know then what a recent study has indicated: Urologists are the most content doctors in practice in the USA.

We were introduced to patient care for the first time in the second year. I can still remember an attractive young woman paraded before the entire class early in the year. She had severe Crohn's disease and was advised to have a total removal of her large intestine. We were asked whether we agreed with the rec-ommendation. None of us could imagine this attractive young lady going through life with a ileostomy and voted against the surgery. Then the professor said: "You have all condemned this young woman to an early demise!" The point was well made!

We were taught what questions we should ask the patient and in what order that should be done. This was known as the "history", which was followed by a physical examination with the patient flat on the examining table, naked, with the sheet pulled up to the level of the lower abdomen to cover his or her genital area. Routine urine and blood tests were done next, f-ollowed by more specific and elaborate tests depending on the nature and severity of the problem. This tradition of history, physical, routine and special laboratory tests dates back a century and continues to this day.

In 1910, Abraham Flexner, a retired school teacher, was commissioned by the Carnegie Foundation to investigate medical "school" teaching in North America. He found much to criticize, that far too many schools at the time existed largely for profit, while only a minority emphasized a scientific basis for the profession as was practiced in Germany. His report was, in fact, high praise and endorsement of what William Osler had been espousing throughout his illustrious professional life, and the institutions with which Osler had any attachment at all, like Johns Hopkins, McGill, and the University of Toronto were singled out for commendation.

Is it time for another Flexner-type review of all medical schools?

Medical school acceptance in North America is highly prized and very competitive today as it was yesterday, but are the best candidates the ones most likely to be picked? If the only criterion considered was scholastic records our schools today might be filled almost completely with Chinese students as they might have been with Jewish students a generation or two ago. Would that be good or bad? We will never know because such an outcome would not be allowed to occur. There are unwritten rules we will never be able to fathom. We can, however, ponder what are the qualities in the applicant that would make him or her more attractive? Medicine should be a calling and two qualities come immediately to my mind as being most important: they are honesty and a capacity for compassion.

These qualities are impossible to measure, at least, with any accuracy. Thus, mistakes are made, and often criticized, but honest efforts are being made to pick the "best" candidates. An applicant with outstanding academic records but with no evidence of acceptable social interaction skills, for example, is less likely to be picked over a candidate with an abundance of obvious social skills. In my lifetime, I have been asked, a number of times, if I could help coach potential applicants. My advice has always been the same over the years: a serious applicant will never accept "no" as an acceptable answer to his application! Memory, though, is capricious! I cannot remember the interview I had as an applicant!

I can remember during my first year in Montreal asking my grade seven teacher, Mrs.Trueman in my first year in Montreal (1946) after our confinement in the war camps whether Harry Truman, the president of the USA would have dropped a nuclear bomb on a city populated by white citizens. I thought it was fair question because, somehow, I connected my new teacher to the president of the USA although their names were spelled slightly differently. Certainly, it was pronounced the same! I remember her stammering without being able to give me an answer.

In grade nine, we were given a vocational guidance questionnaire at the end of which was the question: Do you have any questions? I wrote down: is it true that if you are a Japanese-Canadian, you cannot become a lawyer? I was sent down to the principal's office and the principal berated me: "We live in a democracy where that kind of thing is just not tolerated. But, it turned out I was more right than the principal. A Japanese-Canadian, in the fifties, might be accepted into law school but that did not mean he would be given a license to practice law. Medicine was more accepting and that's where I turned.

Medical school and post-graduate training are expensive undertaking for our society as the fees charged to the student cover only a fraction of the cost, about ten percent according to a number of studies. Thus, every student should give something back to the society that has supported him or her. I said this once to a collection of students. "But," they replied, "it is not us who do not wish to work here. It's the government that decides how many are acceptable, and the number of slots are few and far between. Deaths, departures or retirement may open up a slot, but not the presence of a willing and available candidate." And, the students were right. Applicants to medical school from outside the country pay higher fees. The larger fee paid by someone from Saudi Arabia, for example, helps with the university budget, and is acceptable if enough doctors are being produced to fill the country's need.

The schooling itself, though, is largely tests of stamina, health, and motivation. Without a strong desire to succeed, success is unlikely, but it is hard to fail with appropriate motivation. Instructions on how to conduct oneself as a professional, on the other hand, is never taught: it is assumed.

The way medicine is practiced, though, changes with new knowledge, innovations, and improved efficiency. My impression is that long and outdated routines that may have served the profession well in the past are slow to be discarded.

For example, in the last half century enormous advances in routine laboratory testing have been made. A dip-stick urinalysis, as an example, can tell us in an instant, and quite accurately, whether there is a bacterial infection as the nitrite band would have turned positive, or whether there is blood in the urine suggesting a possible tumor or stone disease, or sugar implying probable diabetes. And, as we all know, an unbelievable number of tests can be done on a few drops of blood. Also, results that used to take days are delivered now in a matter of hours.

Perhaps the time has come to re-think the traditional way medicine is practiced. Maybe the doctor should look first at the urine and blood results which could be done before he even sees his patient. If the C-reactive protein score in the blood sample is abnormally high, for example, the doctor would be alerted to the fact that he is dealing with a patient whose body is fighting an inflammation somewhere in his body, someone who has a potentially serious illness, in other words, and not someone with a stress related issue. The C-reactive protein, in other words, is like the sedimentation rate that measures how quickly red blood cells separate from the serum. The "sed" rate is still used but was more popular a generation or two ago, often to gauge how sick a patient with tuberculosis might be. It is a measure of the body's reaction to insult or injury. We need more tests like that to help us distinguish "organic" from stress related issues.

DNA analysis of blood or sputum is not yet routine, but it is bound to become so. The results should tell us if a particular patient has a predisposition to a specific disorders or even the presence of actual disease in certain instances. DNA analysis on tissue sample can ascertain prognosis far more accurately than any other test we have today. Already, the DNA analysis of a thyroid cancer, as one example, can tell us if we are dealing with a relatively benign or a seriously malignant form of the disease. These tests are very expensive today, but the cost will come down for certain. Consider the tumbling cost of information available on the internet.

The traditional "history" has a pre-planned order. Questions about past illnesses come first, followed by queries of known allergies, familial predisposition to different illnesses, then history of the present illness, and finally, a review of all systems. Then comes the physical examination that implicates palpation, percussion and auscultation. Gentle, but firm fingertips feel for normal and abnormal structures, tapping for sound distinguishes solid from hollow organs, and the stethoscope detects normal or abnormal body sounds from the heart, lung, bowel and even arteries.

The physical is done with the patient lying on the examining table with discreet covering of intimate body parts. I was chastised early in my practice for doing the rectal examination with men standing up and bent forward with their hands on the examining table rather than by lying on his side, curled up. That was not a discreet position, I was told, not respectful of the dignity of man. But, I argued, the rectal examination of the prostate is done to test for hard lumps and symmetry of the gland. How can you determine symmetry or asymmetry with the patient lying on his side? It is much easier to make this assessment standing right behind the patient. Dignity be damned, I argued, and I continued to do the rectal examination with men standing and bent forward - throughout my career!

When patients are sick enough to require hospital care or need an invasive procedure, the privilege to admit a patient to a particular hospital is limited to doctors "on staff," although a patient may be admitted from the Emergency room. Such patients come under the care of the doctor "on call." He may then be "booked" for surgery.

A patient booked for surgery is never cancelled in the USA. Why would an activity that generates income for the hospital be cancelled? Such cancellations occur regularly in Canada. The common excuse is "no beds." No beds is euphemism for "no nurses" and there are insufficient number of nurses hired so that the hospital budget is not strained. The nursing budget is a significant part of the hospital budget. The easiest way to cut expenses is to have less nurses and, thus, do less procedures. The explanation "Sorry – no bed!" is more acceptable than "Sorry, we're over budget!"

The doctors and the patients can rant and rave but nothing will happen unless the patient is a big-time hospital supporter or donor. The budget, in Canada, is the top priority! On the whole, though, the Canadian Medicare system is far better than what exists in the USA. After all, no matter how extensive the private insurance coverage a patient might have in the USA, it will be depleted by a series of serious health problems. That cannot happen in Canada. That alone makes the Canadian plan better. You get a better night's sleep knowing that a health problem in the family is not ever going to bankrupt you.

At one time I thought I would try my hand at medical fiction. My draft of the "no bed" issue went as follows:

"No bed? What do you mean... no bed?"

"It means, sir, we cannot do your operation to-day. There is no bed to accommodate you after the surgery."

"I'll sleep on a cot..."

"No, sir. No bed doesn't mean there are no hospital beds. There are plenty of hospital beds. It's just that we can't use them."

"Why not?"

"Because there are no nurses to service them."

"Ahh, so it's not "no beds" it's really "no nurses.""

"That is correct, sir."

"And why do we not have the nurses?"

"I can't answer that, sir. You will have to talk to administration."

"This hospital, miss, got me to come down here a few weeks ago for a battery of tests. I had to have a cardiogram, a chest x-ray, blood tests, and urine tests. I was interrogated by young doctors as well as by an anaesthesiologist-in-training. They got me to drink two bottles of some god-awful liquid that turned my crap into pure water. And, they ordered me not to put a drop of food or liquid in my body after midnight, last night ... And now, you tell me it was all for nothing."

"I'm very sorry, sir."

"Sorry? Sorry just doesn't cut it, miss. I bet if I were the prime minister, a bed would be found."

"I suspect you are right, sir."

"And, I suspect there has been no public announcement that the hospital emergency room has been closed."

"Why would you expect that, sir?"

"The hospital cannot look after me, but it can look after disasters brought to the emergency room."

"You have a point, sir."

"Damn right! The hospital cancels my surgery but participates in a grand deception suggesting it can handle disasters brought to its door."

"I do sympathize..."

"You're sorry. I'm sure you are sorry. I bet my doctor is sorry too. Everybody is sorry. Who's not sorry?"

"I think everybody is sorry, sir."

"No, miss, I don't think so. I don't think the administration is sorry.

"I'm sure the administration is very sorry, sir."

"Young lady, I applaud your mislaid loyalty. But, just think about it. What is the role of administration in a publicly funded institution? What makes them look good? Let me tell you. It's coming in on budget. And how do you come in on budget? You restrict services. You hire less nurses. That's how!"

"I never thought of it that way. You may have a point, sir."

"I have no business complaining to you, miss. But why is it you and not someone from administration who comes to tell me the bad news? Do they think I'm less likely to complain if they send an attractive young lady to give me the bad news?"

Health care fiction might be fun to try!

You can choose your own physician or medical specialist in

Canada. He or she is not assigned to you as might be the case in some country. But, how do you choose the best doctor?

Let me relate a true, personal, story.

On an afternoon in April 2007 a package was delivered to my office located on the 6th floor Surgical Wing of the Royal Victoria, then on Pine Avenue in Montreal, a teaching hospital of McGill University. When I opened the large air-bubbled envelope there was a handsome framed certificate inside indicating that I was picked as one of the "best doctor" in my specialty.

At the time I was seeing a hundred patients a week and working ten hours or more every working day. I considered the recognition to be nothing more than a minor nuisance and an unwanted disturbance. I hung the certificate on the wall of my office, nevertheless, among pictures of my children and grandchildren. I had not heard of any organization called "Best Doctors" and I had no idea how reputable it was.

A short time later, I had a visitor to my office – a financial advisor! He saw the certificate on the wall and remarked: "That is quite a singular honor. I know of only one other doctor in the city with the same certificate."

I have since discovered that "Best Doctor" is selected by colleagues who are asked: "Which doctor would you choose to look after you or your loved one if you needed a doctor in this specialty or that..."

"Best Doctors," it turned out, was started in 1989 by Harvard medical professors and it was a reputable organization that tried to match patients to the best possible medical care for patients who sought it.

Why then was I chosen when I have never been asked who I would pick? Certainly it was not because I had an academic appointment at McGill University, nor because I served a period in an administrative role, that of "Program Director" in Urology because under those criteria many doctors qualified. Could it be because I authored a few books on health care for the general public? (Private Parts, The Prostate, Zen in Action). Perhaps... but more likely, it was because doctors surveyed felt I would honestly do what was best for them. Most doctors I know and admire are like that: I would trust them with my life. And I have, as I required cardiac by-pass surgery in 2008.

What is it that makes certain doctors special? If I were to talk to doctors selected as "best doctors" will I be able to determine what set them apart? Maybe there was material here for another book!

My plan was simple and straight-forward. I will call the "Best Doctor" organization in Boston and its satellite branch in Toronto and ask them to give me the names of the doctors in different specialties. I will interview them with pre-set questions:

Why do you think you were selected by your colleagues?

What makes you different from your fellow practitioners?

In what order would you prioritize skill, knowledge, and compassion?

What common problems do you look after?

What preventative measures do you encourage? Are there prophylactic advice you consider foolish?

Do you pay attention to practice guidelines? Are there diagnostic tests you consider a waste of time?

What therapeutic measures do you favor? Are there treatments you consider nonsensical?

My goodness, the book appeared to be writing itself. Then, I encountered a major roadblock. The "Best Doctor" organization refused to release to me the names of doctors on their list. I was incredulous.

"But you send your appointee an impressive certificate designed for public display. You don't send them a confidential note to be filed away in a secret filing cabinet. It doesn't make sense that you can't release the names to me."

"Sorry, but that's our policy."

Umm, is the reason for the policy commercially motivated? Do they profit by suggesting the appropriate doctor? Are they a "for-profit" organization?

"If I were to suggest a few names, can you tell me if they are on your list?"

"Sorry, the answer is no."

My thoughts of material for another book came to an abrupt end. I did ask a number of doctors, though, what characteristics they considered most important in a doctor: knowledge, skill or compassion. I got interesting answers, but my brother, a retired general surgeon gave me the best answer.

"It depends what you're seeing the doctor for," he said. "If it's a family doctor you need, I would pick the one who will make himself or herself most available to me. If I needed major surgery, I would go with the one who has the reputation for being the most skilled. I wouldn't care if he or she is or was widely known to be a S.O.B."

The Hospital

In 2015, a brand new university teaching hospital was opened in Montreal. It was meant to replace five crumbling institutions associated with McGill university, namely: the Royal Victoria Hospital, the Montreal General Hospital, the Royal Chest Hospital, the Montreal Children's Hospital, and the Montreal Neurological Institute. Along the way the Montreal General hospital decided not to close down although its mission was changed somewhat, and the Montreal Neurological Institute decided to delay its closure and its move to the new location - indefinitely.

The new, largely white building complexes in the west end

of the city resemble, to some degree, perhaps only in color, the architecture of the University of Montreal, the Cormier creation, as though the two were meant to be sister institutions. The multi-million dollar project was the brain-child (I think) of Pediatricians of the Montreal Children's Hospital who feared their hospital was at risk of being gobbled up by the expanding Ste. Justine's hospital, the Pediatric teaching hospital associated with the Francophone University of Montreal. Montreal is a bilingual city, more French-speaking than English-speaking, population-wise, although every hospital in the city is supposed to offer services in both languages. In reality, each hospital is more French-speaking or more English-speaking and services in the "other" language are often less than completely satisfactory. Furthermore, it is debatable whether the city required a brand new super-hospital at this time, or two new super-hospitals as it turned out because McGill could not have a new teaching hospital without the University of Montreal getting one too.

When is there a need in any community for a new hospital? Certainly when the old one cannot physically accommodate the new technology like the immense robotic surgery paraphernalia, the lithotripter (stone crushing machine), the PET scanner, the radio-therapy equipment, et cetera, that all take up a lot of space. The modern hospital will need the space to house these new tools, as well as access to more electricity to power them. There may be a need, as well, for a roof that doesn't leak and plumbing that is reliable. Were the "crumbling buildings" beyond repair as often argued or simply unfixable with in-house repair? Could a whole pavilion been closed, for example, fixed, and restored to full function? Would that have cost more or less than a new hospital? Was that ever seriously considered?

No doubt, the idea of a brand-new, mammoth, modern hospital is very attractive to many people. But, what about studies that have shown that hospitals that exceed five hundred beds become inefficient – that five hundred bed hospitals that compete with one another provide the best services. The contention that 500 bed hospitals work best jives with common sense. In the smaller hospitals there are no mysterious hierarchy of power that plague the giant hospital, referral patterns are straightforward, everybody "on staff" knows exactly what can be done and what cannot. It is like suggesting that a community served by one giant supermarket might be worse off than one wherein a number of lesser stores compete for the same customers. Western society was built on healthy competition. That applies to health care as much as to any other aspects of life.

When the Royal Victoria Hospital and the Montreal General Hospital were competing institutions in Montreal, for example, there was a widely circulated anecdote. A rich dowager specified in her will that should she fall ill and could not express her wishes she wanted care at one institution (let's say the Royal Victoria), that no expenses were to be spared in her care but, upon her demise, what was left of her estate was to be donated to the other hospital (the Montreal General).

It is not clear to me who was responsible for the decision but the new super-hospital is supposed to be for tertiary care only. Health care is supposed to be primary, secondary, or tertiary. Who makes the distinction? I am not certain I can. If I have a tummy ache am I supposed to go for primary care somewhere else? What if the reason for the pain is stomach cancer? Tertiary-care-only policy is not the custom of renowned cancer centers in the USA. Is it practiced anywhere? It must be but I don't know where. I asked the former head of Urology at Sloan-Kettering what he does when he is referred a minor problem – a man who needs surgery for a hydrocele, a benign fluid collection in the scrotum, for example. "I accept it," he said. "If you don't accept the small stuff, you don't get referred the big case," he said.

There have been a number of unfortunate scandals associated with the McGill mega project. Major construction projects in Montreal have traditionally been associated with scandal. I have heard people in the trade tell me that no major projects get done in Montreal or Quebec, for that matter, without an envelope slipped under the table. Still, twenty-five to thirty million dollars that cannot be accounted for seems outrageously scandalous.

Let me relate a few anecdotes I associate with the mega-hospital project.

Early on, we had a visit from one of the prime movers of the project.

"We have narrowed potential sites for the new hospital to five," he said, "but, I cannot divulge the sites because we cannot afford to have land speculation."

"So," I said, "we have people who know and people who don't know, and you are asking those of us who don't know to support those who do know. Does that not defy human nature?"

It was not a popular comment.

The first CEO appointed for the project was Hugh Scott, a cardiologist. I remember serving on a McGill research board with Hugh many years ago. He, more than any other doctor, wanted no financial contributions from big pharma to help our effort. He strongly felt that money from the pharmaceutical industry would corrupt our mission. Others did not fully agree with him, but Hugh, even then, argued his case eloquently. I also remember an address Hugh made to a huge audience at the Royal Victoria.

"I finally found out what CEO stands for," he said. "It stands for Career Ending Opportunity."

Scott served his time and was replaced by Dr. Arthur Porter, a radio-oncologist. I had met Dr. Porter on one of the prostate cancer meetings held regularly in Whistler, British Columbia. Dr. Porter had an enviable reputation as a polished speaker. Under Dr. Porter the new McGill University hospital came into being. Scandal surfaced when inquisitive reporters uncovered millions of dollars that could not be accounted for, including not one but two Bentleys assigned to him. Arthur Porter fled to Panama where he died of lung cancer before he could face an inquiry and justice before the court.

I was referred a patient who was on the committee that picked Arthur Porter.

"You knew that Arthur Porter did not have a stellar reputation in Detroit," I said. "What made you all select him?"

"Let me tell you," said my patient, as he settled into his chair. "Let us suppose we advertise for a new position – CEO of MUHC (McGill University Health Centre). Forty people apply for the job. One of them happens to be Arthur Porter. You would have picked him."

"Wow!"

My guess, in hindsight, is that they needed someone who was willing to cheat, to lie, to break a few laws. They recognized that a truly honest man could not get the job done. At least, that is what I think.

As I have indicated before, I am not a fan of mammoth hospitals. Smaller hospitals that compete with one another is what I think works best for any community. And, as I have also indicated earlier, a tent can be a hospital if the roof doesn't leak and there is sufficient access to electricity.

While I am in this critical mode, let me also lash out on what I think is wrong with health care delivery in this country. The system is geared to reward quantity over quality, treatment over prevention, and copies over originals. Let me elaborate.

A doctor working under the government Medicare scheme

is rewarded for the number of patients he has seen or the number of procedures he has carried out, regardless whether his diagnosis or treatment was correct, incorrect or inappropriate. The presumption that every doctor is equally competent and caring is naive to say the least. In the open market fees will vary to reflect the reputation established. This may be inappropriate, on occasions but, with time, should be self-correcting.

Under the Canadian government scheme, if the first visit warrants a second visit and more tests, the doctor is further rewarded. The system rewards "creative billing" over "better care." The doctors are doing piece-work and the emphasis is on how many patients he can process in a unit of time. Then, the doctor is instructed to prescribe a generic drug over the original. The generic drugs are every bit as good as the originals, in quality, but the firms that make them have not spent one penny on the drug's development. It takes tens of millions of dollars to produce one new drug fit for public consumption. Companies that produce the generics have not spent one penny doing this and thus should be allowed to charge manufacturing costs plus profit. That does not come to the kind of price charged for the drugs. The profit margin for generic drug makers is astronomical. The government itself should get into the business of making the generic drugs.

And, as I have indicated before, I believe that as doctors are largely products of dollars collected from the citizens of the land there should be a responsibility for them to give back to the community. In fact they do with the taxes they pay over their lifetime, but not if they move out the country shortly after graduation. Elsewhere I have indicated that it is largely the government that decides the number of professionals that should be licensed per geographical location. Might there not be room for a little competition? Why is there so much competition to get into medical school, and so little for a job assignment? Free enterprise has worked pretty well in the western world, after all.

We should find a better way to pay our doctors. I have given it some thought and I will indicate what I think is appropriate and reasonable. First though, let me say that doctors are not the only people in our society where productivity and reward are not always in accord. What about our bankers, our business men, our athletes, our actors, our poets? How can bankers (in the USA) go beg the president for help at the time of the financial crisis travelling in their private jets? Why should athletes get astronomical rewards for what they might do? Like everybody else should they not be rewarded for what they have done? Everybody's income tax statement, especially if they are paid by public funds, should be made an accessible public document, cheaters should face fines and public humiliation. High tax payers should be proud of their contribution to their country.

Many of the super- rich are accumulating wealth without an appropriate contribution to society. Their hired hands find ways to avoid taxes. Does that make them innocent? To my way of thinking, many of the "super-rich" are behaving like the French aristocrats at the time of the French revolution. Is there not a possibility of a similar revolution? The threat seems real enough to me as the top 1% are getting richer and richer at the expense of the vast majority who struggle more and more just to stay afloat. Isn't that a formula for civil unrest? There are accomplished wealthy people, like Bill Gates or Warren Buffet, for example, who are trying to redress this issue, but not all super-rich people are as considerate. I believe that unless we resolve this problem of wealth reallocation, we are inviting World War III – a violent civil war! Are the antics of Donald Trump a prelude to this? Why does he not divulge his tax statements? What can he be hiding?

Let me get back to health care.

How can I advise our citizens to best navigate the complex problem of obtaining the best medical care. Health care for everybody, including seniors, involves five levels of activity. In recent times a sixth category has emerged, that is, end-of-life, or palliative care, so there are now six levels of activity. They are:
- Health promotion
- Specific prevention
- Early Diagnosis and Treatment
- Disease limitation
- Rehabilitation
- Palliative care

Health Promotion

What constitutes Health Promotion for the general public, including the senior citizen? Health care guidelines should be prepared by professionals, combining the input from government, university, and community. They should be simple documents for widespread free distribution. The document should indicate what constitutes acceptable care for different age categories. How often should regular visits to the physician occur when there are no problems: should it be every six months, annually, or what? What information should every patient bring to these meeting: perhaps a list of his medications or, should it be more than that? Should he have a summary of his previous hospitalizations, or previous health problems? What standard laboratory tests are indicated for different age categories? Do we have such a list? We are entering the era of artificial intelligence, and a wearable monitor, looking like a wrist-watch, can record and transmit a cardiogram to the treating doctor.

Other monitors can test blood sugar level. Serum salt levels and other readings, without a needle puncture, are about to become routine, I suspect. What about routine ultrasound examinations of the abdomen and pelvis? CT examination of the lungs has been discussed. What about routine blood chemistries: in the absence of problems how often should they be done? Should problems with sexual orientation constitute expenses covered by our tax dollars?

When I think back to my own years in practice I am certain I gave more time and consideration to those patients who came for their routine office visit with clear documentations. I am sure there was an unconscious effort on my part to reward those who tried to make my life easier. How can you treat someone who shows you the list and dosages of the medications he takes in the same way as another who can't remember three of the eight pills he takes?

What are the currently acceptable screening tests? Why are they not made more mandatory? What kind of information on nutrition and supplements should be provided to the population at large to ensure a healthy life? Should supplements be provided without cost if the physician deems that his patient is not getting them? If that were to happen, does the country come out ahead or behind in terms of total overall costs? Do people who pay attention to healthy habits actually help the economy of his country? Could it not be more widely publicized that a twenty minutes exercise, like a walk every day can improve health and lengthen life?

Perhaps it can and should go further. How much money is actually necessary for an acceptable lifestyle in our society? Could that or should that be provided to families failing to meet that standard? What "strings," if any, need be attached? Is the country rich enough to offer it as a gift? I actually think it is! Should it be a loan? What should be the rate at which it is paid back if it is a loan? Can it be repaid with volunteer work? Why not? How can it be ascertained that financial help will not be used to support drug or alcohol abuse? (I know that student loans were issued, at times, to those who didn't need it. I know students who invested it for profit.) There are always risks with government hand-outs. If the punishment for misrepresentation and deception are substantial, though, the scheme can work or be made to work. I think Norway has done that with its north sea oil wealth. Kudos to Norway!

Smoking must still be taboo. Excess calories are bad for everybody regardless of age. So is excess alcohol. Exercise, a positive outlook, a genuine concern for others, laughter, and a sense of community are all decidedly good. How can they be made the way of the land? The older citizens may need gentle reminders of these "facts of life" from time to time, again and again. Bad habits are easily acquired even in the older population. Has anyone in a hurry ever accomplished more? Age alone should not be an excuse to stop being active in mind and body. Look at our expanding lifespan and look at what is still taking lives.

Good nutrition, a place to exercise, and a place to socialize must all be made accessible to every citizen. The biggest threat to a longer life in western society is processed food. Like the cigarette makers of the last generation, excess sugar is shortening lives but that matters little to the makers of processed food and sweets. Profit is foremost to them even if they are killing the very hand that is feeding them.

It is time for a stronger stance by the community and the health care leaders. The pitch for unhealthy food is organized and led by determined people. It must be countered by equally strong-minded people who treasure life over momentary gratification. Sweetened drinks, carbonated or not could be heavily taxed, for example, if that would discourage them. I doubt that punishment for sweets will work! Rewards for good behavior has always worked better than punishment for bad behavior.

Thus, membership to gyms, pools, or meditation classes should not only be encouraged but made free and readily available to the senior citizen, perhaps to all citizens. Trainers should serve a wider segment of the population. And, as working on crosswords, puzzles, or other mental challenges have been shown to lengthen life as well as contribute to well-being, these activities must not only be encouraged but be made more routine and mandatory. Children in school are monitored regarding education, nutrition, and exercise. We must do the same for the senior citizen, perhaps all citizens.

I wonder if current-day medical students learn about rickets only as a historical phenomenon, like smallpox, beri-beri and scurvy – wiped out by vaccination, vitamin B and vitamin C, respectively. Rickets is due to a deficiency in vitamin D and affected children develop soft bones and become horribly bow-legged. The disease can occur in adults as well and is called osteomalacia. Vitamin D deficiency occurs when there is inadequate exposure to sunshine. Normally, sunshine on skin produces vitamin D which helps the body absorb calcium and phosphorus both necessary for normal bone development and bone health. When there is insufficient exposure to sunshine the deficit can be corrected with vitamin D supplements. One 400 International unit capsule per day is all that is necessary to ensure healthy bones.

Rickets was not uncommon in Montreal less than a century ago. It was wiped out by Dr. Charles Scriver and Arnold Steinberg (who became Chancellor of McGill). Together the two men convinced the largest grocery chain of the day, Steinberg's, to add vitamin D to the milk it sold at its stores. That did the trick! It is a striking example of how good science and good citizens can change the health of a community.

Health promotion can and should be encouraged as a national objective. The government can become more involved in this. I suspect that if the ideal body weight for the different ages were to be more widely publicized, more people will strive to achieve that objective. The BMI may be the more important figure for health care professionals, but the simple measurement of weight is sufficient to encourage changes in the right direction.

Specific Prevention

Protective immunization has an important role to play to ensure good health. Vaccination against "shingles," for example, should be made mandatory for everybody regardless of age. Shingles is caused by the herpes zoster virus and is characterized by a painful skin eruption and pain along the course of the involved sensory nerves. Immunization against this virus is relatively recent but can be highly effective. Annual vaccination against influenza should be routine, even when it is found, at times, to be of questionable effectiveness one year compared to another. Supplemental vitamin D capsules, and Calcium tablets should also be made routine in a temperate country like Canada to lessen the risk of osteoporosis and osteomalacia due to insufficient exposure to sunshine. Denosumab (Prolia) injections twice a year to prevent osteoporosis in post-menopausal women is becoming routine as it should.

What about osteoporosis in men? Certainly older men who are not doing weight-bearing exercises regularly are at risk for developing osteoporosis. A bone density study could and should be done on all senior citizens on a regular basis, perhaps every three years. Men on androgen deprivation therapy for prostate cancer have to be checked for osteoporosis more frequently, perhaps annually, and treated for inevitable osteoporosis from their treatment. Denosumab is the mandatory drug of choice.

Vaccination against herpes, shingles, and hepatitis is appropriate for all citizens, including senior citizens. Vaccination of young girls and boys against condyloma accuminata is going to have an impact on cervical cancer development in women. Why there were objections to this recommendation in some quarters is baffling. The HPV vaccine, called Gardisil-9, will reduce or eliminate the risk of developing cervical cancer. The story behind that is interesting. Cervical cancer was found to be exceedingly uncommon, in fact, unheard of in Roman Catholic nuns. Could it be because of sexual abstinence in this population and, sexual abstinence meant elimination of exposure to condyloma. The hypothesis, it turned out, was right on!

More controversial, perhaps, is hormone replacement therapy for men and women. There was a time when virtually every woman after menopause was advised supplemental estrogen and progesterone. I encouraged it in my practice although most prescriptions were prepared by the gynecologists and family practitioners. This was called hormone replacement therapy and contributed to a younger body, a better sex life, and reduced risks of urinary tract infections. Then, reports surfaced that the risk of developing breast cancer was enhanced. Although the risk was not high, most women and their doctors stopped hormone replacement therapy. Recently, though, it has been determined that the risk of breast cancer for women on estrogen and progesterone (the hormone replacement therapy) was much less worrisome than originally reported and the advantages of hormone replacement far exceeded the disadvantages. In addition to reduced risks of bladder infections, and enhanced sex-life, supplemental estrogens is thought to reduce the risk of developing Alzheimer's disease as well. I believe post- menopausal women will be put back on the hormones as I think they should.

Andropause in men remains a less certain entity. It seemed reasonable to expect that older men might stop or reduce their normal production of testosterone. And, many studies have shown exactly that. A lower testosterone reading meant less libido, less aggressiveness, less muscle mass, and a lesser sex life. Why not hormone-replacement-therapy for men? The concern, of course, was prostate cancer. Giving men testosterone will surely increase their risk of developing prostate cancer, will it not? Only in recent times has it been determined that this presumption was incorrect. Giving men testosterone, especially if their readings were low did not, in fact, increase the risk of developing prostate cancer. This determination is attributed largely to doctor Abraham Morgentaler, originally from Montreal but now associated with Harvard and Boston. Of course, if prostate cancer was already present, testosterone administration will enhance the growth and spread of the disease.

Hormone replacement therapy has become increasingly more popular in recent times for men. Usually, the bio-available testosterone level is measured in the blood sample taken in the morning, between nine and eleven. Readings under 3.5 is considered low. Oral preparations of the drug are non-existent, but preparations rubbed on skin (Androjel), as a skin patch (Testim), or as a nasal inhalation (Natesto) are available. An injectable form of the drug (Delatestryl) is still the most economical. Testing for the hormone levels and prescribing testosterone in one form or another is not quite like testing for diabetes and offering insulin. Often, men will report favorable results even when the tests show no changes and no response when the laboratory results indicate that they should be responding. There is no explanation for that.

In addition to an enhanced sex life and more energy, muscle power should be enhanced. If prostate cancer was not a problem, the only negative reaction to the testosterone administration might be an extra aggressiveness that is seen in some men. Of course, if prostate cancer is present, diagnosed or not, testosterone administration will enhance the growth of the malignancy and spread the disease.

I have prescribed testosterone to men not just for rejuvenating a dwindling sex life but to enhance their diminishing muscle power or energy. In general, I am pleased with the results but remain puzzled why the responses and the blood results are not always in accord. That is to say, the hormone level may be low and the response to testosterone administration negligible in one candidate while another will report marked effect without the blood results showing the corresponding results. I have no explanation for that.

There have been no comparable products for loss of libido in women. Testosterone will enhance female libido, but will also grow a moustache and no woman will accept that. Recently, though, a very low dose testosterone preparation called Tefina has been promoted to enhance libido without unwanted side effects. Whether it will work without side effects remains to be seen. There was also a recent release of a medication touted as a "Viagra for women." The pill, called Addyi (flibanserin) did not live up to expectations.

For both senior men and women, the often repeated established recommendations still apply. Don't smoke, don't drink excessively, weigh yourself and lose weight if necessary, exercise regularly, cultivate a circle of good friends, meditate, and remain optimistic. Is it not getting repetitive?

Early Diagnosis and Treatment

Early diagnosis of an illness and appropriate treatment is what medical practice is all about. That is what every doctor is expected to do and he does it by arranging regular visits even when his patients are well, and extra visits when he or she is not well. As a patient you can make the visit more meaningful by presenting yourself with a carefully prepared document that summarizes your medical history, lists the medications you take on a regular basis, your allergies, if you have any, as well as a summary of the more serious health events in your life. Anyone who presents to the doctor with such a document is likely to get far better care than someone whose past is a blank. Each visit is meant to ascertain an early diagnosis of a malady if something is amiss, and appropriate care if there is a problem.

Treatment is always designated resuscitative, medical or surgical. Another category might be added to this. It might be called "Emerging modalities of treatment" and include immunotherapy and stem cell treatment. These modalities have not yet become standard therapies but I have no doubt that they will become so.

Practice guidelines can be helpful to both patients and doctors. Why can't we have more of them? Remember, though, that guidelines should and must change with time. What are the guidelines I am thinking about? I think there should be routine tests for different age categories. At what age should a routine cardiogram be started, for example. What if there is a family history of heart disease? When should a stress cardiogram be done? What are the indications for an echo study of the heart? When is a stress echo indicated? What should be the routine blood tests done on someone fifty years of age? What changes should be made because he or she is now sixty, or seventy? Should a routine chest x-ray be done? When should it be a chest tomogram? The listing of appropriate tests for different age categories seems most appropriate: who would argue against it! I am unaware that such documents exist! Why don't we have them? Does medical practice change so much and so often that they cannot be kept up-to-date? Personally, I do not think that is the case. If practice guidelines were to be stated in black and white, would it lead to more medical-legal issues because the doctor chose to ignore them? Could that be the reason why guidelines seem so scarce? Guidelines available to both patients and doctors should make health-care safer and better in my estimation.

In the previous section I described the recognized common causes of death in Canada. Become aware of them and adopt measures to assure early diagnosis of any disorder, especially those with life threatening potential. For example, every senior citizen should have an annual electro-cardiogram, perhaps a stress cardiogram as well as an echo cardiogram. If the heart-beat is irregular, a consultation with a cardiologist is mandatory, and a recommendation for a blood thinner routine. There are many blood thinners besides the traditional heparin and Coumadin. Newer drugs require much less monitoring, but is the one prescribed appropriate for the person's unique situation? The cardiologist should be able to convince the patient why the medication he has prescribed might be the best one for his or her particular situation. Regular low dose chest tomograms may be the only way an early diagnosis of lung cancer can be ascertained. Can our society afford such a measure? Before debating the issue we must ask the question: Which costs more: regular low dose chest tomograms for everybody and early lobectomy for cure or late diagnosis and total lung excision followed by chemo and radiotherapy that is often unsuccessful.

I suspect the patient who had the chest tomogram, an early diagnosis of lung cancer and curative surgery would have rung up a lesser cost than the unscreened patient whose advanced disease necessitated unsuccessful surgery. Similarly, annual PSA (prostate specific antigen) blood test and annual digital rectal exam should assure early diagnosis of prostate cancer, a likely cure and lesser cost than his twin who is diagnosed late with metastatic disease and requires hormone therapy, palliative radiotherapy and chemotherapy. Regular colonoscopy should assure early diagnosis of colon and rectal cancer and, in the long run, cost less than unsuccessful treatment for advanced disease.

We have, presently, no screening tests to assure early diagnosis of pancreatic cancer, leukemia, lymph node cancers, ovarian cancers, and many other cancers. Undoubtedly, it is the lack of good screening tests or the failure to carry them out when they do exist that makes cancer the number one killing disease of our civilization. It makes no sense to cut down on the sugar, exercise regularly, meditate - and lose your life to a delayed diagnosis of a curable cancer.

When the early diagnosis of lung cancer is missed – who is at fault? Is it the patient who did not ask for a chest tomogram? Is it the doctor who did not order it? Is it the health professionals in government who don't insist upon practice guidelines? Should not advanced countries in the western world have such guidelines?

Let's get back to the subject of early diagnosis and treatment.

Treatment is always designated as resuscitative, curative, (medical or surgical) or palliative. As already suggested, I believe there are two emerging modalities of treatment; namely, immunotherapy and stem cell therapy that should be added to this. They are not yet fully established to count as legitimate treatment but that time will come.

Disease Limitation, Rehabilitation, and End of Life Care completes the format.

Anyone with a clear idea of this format, which I have repeated again and again, should have a clear understanding of what health care is all about.

Health care may be compromised because there is no access to doctors or other health care professionals. This has become a problem under Medicare in Canada with family doctors having enough patients under their care to want or need more. Would nurse practitioners be the solution to this problem? If there are not enough doctors to fill the need, nurse practitioners seem a logical solution. But, is it? Is it like suggesting that since there are not enough surgeons to do the job, let's have the family doctors do the surgery? We do need to better define what could or should be done and by whom. In rural Ontario, nurse-practitioners have done and continue to do a phenomenal job filling the need for primary care. Should that service be expanded across the country? Or, should we consider graduating more doctors? As the doctor population becomes more and more female, as is the case, and with established statistics that indicate women spend less years in practice, it's common sense that we will have to graduate more doctors.

Community wide vaccination should be done by nurses or, perhaps, by pharmacists. Can deciding who needs what kind of care, or triage, be done by trained personnel? Can it be done by nurses? Do we need doctors to do that? I think that what is required is on the job training. Experience may not teach us everything, but it is what best prepares us for surprises. A competent operation is one with experience. Experience can prepare us even for what has never been seen or done before. One of the recurring complaints about health care in Canada is the long wait at the hospital Emergency Room. Can we not stream-line triage? Maybe recently-retired-professionals can be lured back to provide this service. A mistake can be deadly, but experienced personnel are the only ones that can do this quickly with a minimum of errors. I am thinking here of retired doctors. If they are alert and want to participate in health care, they can fill the bill.

Life threatening health issues in the elderly population are no different from those in younger people, but lesser health problems may occur more often in older people. These problems include the following:

1. Osteoarthritis. This is often called the "wear and tear" arthritis. It will never be seen in anyone in his twenties or thirties. But, starting in the forties and beyond, people who have overworked their joints may have ground down the protective material on the surface of joints. It's not unlike a door hinge that has lost its lubrication and the continued opening and closing grinds down the metal surfaces of the joint. In the very worst situation a short course of cortisone-type drugs are prescribed. In less severe conditions, anti-inflammatories, like acetaminophen (Tylenol) and Aspirin are prescribed. In severe cases, joint replacement surgery becomes necessary.

2. Vision, hearing, smell and taste are all faculties that diminish with time. The capacity to imagine, invent, compose, and hypothesize are all considered domains of the young. No senior citizen gets awarded a research grant for original research. Too bad! The one capacity that defies this deterioration is wisdom. We don't get smarter as we age but we can and do get wiser.

3. Accidents and falls occur with more serious consequences as we get older. Remember, the most common cause of accidents in the elderly are area rugs and slippery bathroom floors.

4. Depression is a problem in 15 to 20% of people over the age of 65. Anti-depressants are readily available to help, but poverty is an equally common problem. The country has the resources to help in this situation, but

we don't implement it as a routine. That is too bad. Let me though, for a moment, make the opposing argument. Why should people who have scrimped and saved over their lifetime to provide for a better retirement be further taxed to help those who were less careful, less frugal? As can be imagined it is not always easy to propose a plan that would be viewed in the same way by different people.

5. Bowel and urinary incontinence are the final indignation. These are usually not isolated problems and there are no simple solutions. Adult diapers, though, are much better than they were a generation ago.

What could improve health care in Canada? To put the remarks in perspective, I need to explain myself more fully. I am a product of the public school system of Quebec and I graduated in 1951 from the quintessential public school of Anglophone Montreal – the High School of Montreal. My classmates were, I think, from the working class with a generous sprinkling of boys of Jewish background. Many of my classmates went on to become doctors, dentists, lawyers, architects, engineers and other professionals. The High School of Montreal was sex segregated and had more than a half a dozen classes of the same grade. Those who took Latin were in the "A" class and those who took advanced math were in the "B" class, and these two classes had most of the students who went on to university. I took Latin and was in the "A" class. I am one of three classmates who became medical doctors. The "B" class also had three students who became medical doctors.

I did an honours course in Psychology in my undergraduate years and applied to the McGill medical school in 1955, the year I earned my Bachelor degree. Acceptance into med school was highly prized then as it is now. Many apply and few were accepted, then as now. I don't know and wonder to this day whether being a scholarship student at the museum of fine arts, by the school run by Arthur Lismer, of the group of seven, contributed in any way towards my acceptance. My marks were okay but not, in my view, exceptional. We went from high school to university in those days, with no college or what is called CGEP in between. I found out that the "Arts" students, working towards a BA, took four courses each year and the "Science" students, working towards a BSc took five. I registered for six courses in year one after finding out, to my astonishment, that there was no extra charge for doing so. The extra course was "Introduction to Greek philosophy," or something close to that, a subject that had captured my fancy at the time. The course was taken by only a handful of students.

I don't remember much of it, but the ancient Greeks were searching for the one substance or the one principle that underlined, or explained, our existence: was it solid, ethereal, or what? Was there a single principle that explained all of humanity? These were questions I brooded about at the time and wasn't university the place to find the answers. The ancient Greeks considered water as the primary substance, then air, and few other candidates, but came up, in fact, with a blank. The search continues to this day for the one theory that can explain everything, from quantum physics to the string theory. These speculations raise as many questions as resolve quandaries, I had come to conclude.

I figured I had to do more than reasonably well in the traditional subjects, like Organic Chemistry and Physics if I was serious about Medicine as a career. It was at about this time, I think, that I discovered to my astonishment that high school Latin was not a prerequisite for med school. I am certain I took

Latin in high school because I thought it was. I did not like Latin, like I did not like French as a subject either, and I abhorred the Japanese language classes during my internment camps years. I don't know why languages were so difficult for me. Maybe it was because I started school in English without being able to speak word of it. I remember wetting my pants because I didn't know how to ask permission to go to the bathroom.

My lowest mark, in my high school matriculation exams was in English composition. To this day I don't know why I scored so badly in high school English. My compositions always earned the comment "Good imagination" but marks were deducted for misplaced commas or errors in conjugation which, in my estimation, were not nearly as important as "flights of fancy." I sneaked a look at compositions by my classmates who had scored higher marks. They were all disgustingly boring in my view. After that, I stopped paying attention to grades as far as English composition was concerned. In my first year at university, English was a compulsory course. We were assigned a tutor, or advisor with whom we met at regular intervals.

My tutor was Louis Dudek, an established author and poet. Professor Dudek liked my compositions and gave me marks I never got in high school. He even took me aside one day and encouraged me to continue writing. He thought I had potential! I have authored three books (four, if this manuscript is ever published) in my lifetime and I am certain it never would have happened without my encounter with Louis Dudek. (I had the opportunity to tell him of his influence on my life years later when he became my patient. He rewarded me with copies of all his books.) In year two of undergraduate studies I took the introductory course in Psychology, like many hundreds, perhaps thousands of other students, as part of my curriculum.

Professor Donald Hebb lectured to an immense, amorphous

class with a microphone at the head of a large auditorium in what was called Moyse Hall. On one occasion, he declared that hypnosis was simply the power of suggestion and that he could put asleep all the students in the auditorium who felt inclined to follow his suggestion. And he did! I felt myself about to fall asleep but, at the last moment, I decided to stay awake as a witness to the event. I was totally impressed with the power of suggestion. (Years later, at a party of medical residents and nurses, I declared that hypnosis was simply powerful suggestion and that I could put asleep anyone who would volunteer to be a subject. Two nurses volunteered against my wildest expectations. I had no choice. I instructed the nurses to open and close their eyes repeatedly and then declared that now they would not be able to open their eyes. The heads of the two nurses slumped forward. I panicked and ordered them to wake up immediately. I, more than anyone else, was astounded at the power of suggestion.

A multiple choice exam was administered at the end of the school year for the course in Introductory Psychology. I came out of the exam setting not knowing whether I had passed or failed, but when the results were posted, as all results were, I found my name the third one from the top. The two names ahead of mine were those of more senior students. I have no idea why I did so well in that course. It might just as well have been a computer glitch. Or, possibly, it was because I read professor Hebb's book "The Organization of Behaviour." It was a fascinating read, and it made a lot of sense to me. It proposed, as an example, that our minds worked to make habits of our behavior. Thus, if we repeated names, like MacDonald, MacLeod, MacNeil, and MacArthur, and came across machine, it will come out as MacHine.

The secret of life lay not in anything we might find in the

physical world (as the Greeks thought) but in determining how the mind functioned. I applied, then, to take the honour's course in Psychology. I thought that it may be my way to get into med school or, failing that, I could consider a career in Psychology. I became friendly with the professors in Psychology, like Wally Lambert, Ronald Melzack (who became an authority on pain), and Dr. Bindra (I never got his first name), who gave me a summer job and encouraged me to pursue a career in Psychology. In the final year of undergraduate studies I was asked if I wanted to become involved in the sensory deprivation experiment for which the university became famous or, more accurately, infamous. It was many years later when I learned that the US Secret Service, the CIA, was financing the research, nominally under the supervision of the chief of Psychiatry, Dr. Ewen Cameron. I never met Dr. Cameron, personally, although he did lecture to our first, or second year medical class on a few occasions. I found him pompous and distant unlike Donald Hebb who was friendly, fascinating, and inspiring. I must mention that I was not the brains running the sensory deprivation experiments, I just did the leg work. I fed the subjects when they said they were hungry, I escorted them to the bathroom, I measured their temperature, their pulse and blood pressure before and after they emerged from isolation. I administered a form of IQ test, as well, before and after their period of sensory deprivation. Each student volunteer was paid $25.00 per day and most lasted two days, on average. (I honestly can't remember if I got paid for the hours I put in. I don't think I did.) The subjects were all male and thought they were in isolation for a much longer time.

A medical student, who later became the chief of Surgery at Sherbrooke University lasted the longest – six days. Another undergraduate student, who became a medical student developed acute psychosis a few years later. I have long wondered whether his participation in the isolation experiment played any causative role. Each volunteer was placed in a cubicle the area size of a single bed mattress, fitted with walls at its edges and a ceiling so low it did not permit the subject to stand. There was a continuous constant humming sound within the chamber. The subject had wire probes on his scalp to measure brain waves, frosted goggles to eliminate vision, cuffs that extended from forearm to beyond fingertips to eliminate touch and feel.

Most subjects so isolated felt they were confined for weeks when they were in isolation for no more than one day. I believe sensory deprivation was a form of torture pioneered by communist countries and western "intelligence" was just catching up. I did not attend any lectures during my final term as I was totally preoccupied with the project. In 1990, a book called "Father, Son and the CIA" by Harvey Weinstein was released. It relates the story of Harvey's father, who became a patient of Dr. Cameron. The care he was supposed to get was turned into obvious abuse. Harvey Weinstein is a McGill medical school graduate who had become a psychiatrist. I admire his courage in writing the book. It is a compelling read.

I must have disappointed my professors in Psychology, though, for picking Medicine over Psychology as a career choice. I was accepted into Medicine in 1955, graduated in 1959, and qualified as a urologist in 1964. I did a Fellowship in Transplantation Biology as I was finishing my training, earned a PhD in Investigative Medicine and was appointed to the university and hospital staff in 1966. I always believed I had a rather uncommon and unique way of looking at problems. As a child my hero was Thomas Edison and my secret ambition was to become an "inventor". I was saddened to learn, decades later, that some of Edison's innovations were the brainchild of Tesla, now appropriately honored by Elon Musk.

Have I had any worthwhile innovative ideas myself that have been recorded in black and white? I can think of a few. My first publication in the scientific literature was in the journal of social Psychology. Textbooks, at the time (1954-55) stated that children acquire racial discrimination as a skill when they are nine years old. I studied the interaction of four and five year old children of diverse ethnic and racial background in a Montreal day-care as my project and I found clear evidence of racial discrimination as a skill in these children.

I asked each child to hand out candies to two of their best friends, then who each one wanted to have in a picture taken of him or her and, finally, which picture each one liked the most after his or her picture was removed. The choices, I argued, had thus to be made in public, in private, and by projection. It became quite apparent to me that these young children were capable of "racial discrimination." That was my research project for an honor's degree in Psychology. My professor (Wally Lambert) rewrote the paper but made me the first author for its publication in the journal of Social Psychology.

Then, as a junior resident in Urology, I explored the possibility of using the entire length of the small intestine as a dialyzing membrane in what was called the "Taguchi loop." The designation was made by Dr. David Saunders, who was then the chief resident in Internal Medicine and who, subsequently, became a gastroenterologist. I remember being asked a number of times how it feels to have a surgical procedure named after you. Then, I reported a way to connect the ureter to the bladder in a rat kidney transplantation model. I tried the technique in a human trial and reported it in the journal of Urology. Argentinian doctors compared the technique to established procedures and reported the technique to be simpler to carry out with better results than other established methods.

The procedure is widely used today and is known as the Taguchi U-stitch. As an academic I have published my share of papers in scientific journals but what I have mentioned here would be my claims to originality.

My professional career was launched in 1966 close to the time Medicare came into being across Canada (1968). Ask any Canadian to-day what he cherishes most about being a Canadian and I know a surprising number of people will say it is his access to quality health care. Canadians are justifiably proud of their healthcare which is universal, extensive, portable, and publicly administered. What that means is that virtually all health problems are covered by the scheme; the coverage will hold even if the first problem led to a second and the second to the third (unlike private insurance in the USA where the patient will be told he has used up his coverage and is now on his own); the coverage will hold even if the candidate moves from one province to another; and the plan will be run by people who are not necessarily doctors or politicians.

Such a plan was the brainchild of the socialist party leader of Saskatchewan, Tommy Douglas, although he was no longer the premier in 1962 when the plan was adopted in the western province. Despite objections from the medical profession and its organization, the Saskatchewan plan was adopted across the country in 1968, a move spear-headed, I think, by justice Emmett Hall, who headed a commission on health care while on his way to becoming a member of the Supreme Court of Canada. There were many heroes responsible for the Medicare programme in Canada but, if we had to narrow the plaudits to two people: the two might be Tommy Douglas and Emmett Hall.

Much later, I would become the urologist of Morris Fish, of the supreme court of Canada. He invited me to Ottawa and I was taken on a tour of the supreme court building along with my son who accompanied me. Later on, I said to Mr. Fish: "Do you not think the legal profession would be improved if it made the search for truth a priority over the search for justice." Cleverly, he replied: "We are moving in that direction."

I started my clinical work in 1966 so I was in practice for two years before Medicare was launched in Quebec. The specialist doctors in Quebec voted to strike, I remember, certain the government scheme would hurt their income. It was only sometimes later that they realized to their astonishment that their income did not suffer at all under Medicare; it may have even increased as there were no unpaid services. At the time about ten to fifteen percent of all bills sent out were never paid. I can certainly attest to that!

The Medicare scheme is universal across the land but controlled provincially. Thus a fee for a particular act may be more in one province than in another. Fees in Quebec were traditionally lower than those in certain other provinces, like Ontario or British Columbia, and for a radical prostatectomy, as an example, just about half of that in British Columbia, although the cost of living in the two provinces was not that different. I don't know why more fuss was not made over this disparity.

Under Medicare doctors do piece work. They get paid for every patient seen, every act carried out. The quality of work is assumed, never really considered. Theoretically a doctor who processed ten patients and made ten wrong diagnosis still earned twice as much as his confrere who saw five patients in the same period of time, all diagnosed and treated properly. The system could count but does not or could not question quality of care.

I did piece-work as a child picking strawberries on a farm in British Columbia, and my mother did piece-work making blouses on her sewing machine when we first came to Montreal.

I associate piece-work with sweat inducing down right drudgery, not something you agree to after more than fifteen years of intensive post-high school education. Furthermore, to qualify as a specialist in Canada an elaborate system of examinations have to be passed at the end of the training period. The pass rate to obtain the coveted credential was, in my time, roughly one in two. Those who failed to qualify could try again the following year or settle for family practice. Those fortunate enough to pass could add FRCS(C) to their name. That meant he or she was a fellow of the royal college of surgeons.

After all these years of training, I don't think doctors should be doing piece-work. It is demeaning! I think they should be salaried with a salary scale that considers a number of factors, like the number of years of post-secondary studies, his or her university and hospital appointment status, years of experience, amount of committee work, papers published, research done, grants received, national and international recognitions, prizes, etc. Recognition for work in the community as well as volunteer work must and should also be considered. This may seem convoluted and complicated but I don't think it is, nor need to be. If we had ten criteria to consider, for example, each one graded one to three, we could have, theoretically, thirty grades. Doctors could and should strive to improve their station or grade. Presently, a surgeon with ten years of experience for a particular procedure and a reputation for doing it well is rewarded exactly the same amount as a novice trying it for the very first time. Is that right or fair?

The volume of work, the rate of complications, patient satisfaction score, outcomes, failures, disasters, should all be part of the score. There can be a parallel private system, but doctors should not be allowed to practice simultaneously in both systems. A complicated but fair pay scale could and should be better than a scheme that simply counts.

Does such a system exist anywhere? I'm not certain it does but why shouldn't another model be tried: despite the convoluted attempts of the health ministers to make the system work in Canada: it is not working! Or, not working well.

It is common knowledge that most countries in the world spend about ten per cent of its GDP (gross domestic product) on health care. Some countries, like the USA, spend considerably more (15.3% in 2006) but the expenditure is by the well-to-do on what is not essential nor for better care, while many less well-to-do citizens are not covered at all by any plan. Canada's expenditure in 2006 was 10% of GDP.

Japan's expenditure the same year was 8.1%. The expenditure on health care in the different countries the same year was as follows: Switzerland 11.3%, France 11%, Germany 10.6%, Belgium 10.3%, Denmark 9.5%, UK 8.4%, Korea 6.4%) Norway, by the way, spent 8.7%, but their conception of health care includes coverage for university education, as one example. Furthermore, Norwegians are among the most content people inhabiting the world, and also, one of the longest living. The world can learn from them. When the country got rich from off-shore oil, the leaders invested wisely rather than pass it on to its citizens as some other countries did. They are reaping the rewards for the prudent action of its leaders.

What I would like to see most, though, are more details of the expenditures: what are the percent expenditures on different aspects of health care in the different countries. What percentage is spent on health promotion, on specific prevention, on diagnosis and treatment, on disease limitation, on rehabilitation, and on palliative care? Only by having comparable figures can we conclude the value of any undertaking. Is life span impacted by health promotion measures, such as better control of sugar in-

take, compulsory exercise, regular measurements of LDL cholesterol, C-reactive protein, and other blood markers? Without
figures, how can we know?

If the six levels of activities that constitute health care
(HEALTH PROMOTION, SPECIFIC PREVENTION, EARLY
DIAGNOSIS AND TREATMENT, DISEASE LIMITATION, RE-
HABILITATION, AND PALLIATIVE CARE) were to be adopted
as the objectives to strive for, we can then ask the different parties
involved in health care what it is doing regarding each of these
objectives. What has the ministry of health in the current government done regarding health promotion or specific prevention, as an example.

We have enough data now to know there is too much sugar
in our daily diet. How can this problem be addressed? Should
there be a tax on sweetened drinks, carbonated or not? Maybe
we can agree to a prudent limit with anything in excess having
to be a sugar substitute. Would that improve sugar intake?
Should good behaviour be rewarded and bad behavior punished?
Should membership to sport clubs become a tax deductible expense? Should yoga and meditation classes become compulsory
or, at least, a tax deductible expense?

Why isn't all recognized immunization compulsory? Should
those who deliberately decline it enjoy the same health care
coverage should they succumb because of the lack of immunization? This may seem exceptionally harsh on those misled by
unscrupulous individuals but, in my opinion, ignorance and
misapplication of science are not the same thing.

In like fashion, we should re-examine the role and responsibility of those appointed to address health care. What, exactly, is
the responsibility of the Minister of Health? What about the
provincial minister of health? Who is responsible for what? We
know what health care is but should we not debate how much

of our resources should be spent on Health Promotion, how much on Specific Prevention, how much on diagnosis and treatment, how much on basic research? We should know, at a minimum, how much we spend compared to other countries.

Recently, in Quebec (2019), hundreds of doctors (GP's and specialists) signed a document forwarded to the ministry suggesting that the government cancel its pay hikes to the doctors and increase the salaries and working conditions for the nurses of the province. Many nurses were asked or forced to take on double shifts as there were insufficient number of nurses to cope with the need. This kind of bureaucratic mess is unacceptable in today's world. Nurses' salaries and working conditions must be comparable and competitive from one province to another, even one country to another.

What is the hierarchy of power in the current system? We have the Minister of Health, appointed by the government in power. What are his responsibilities? Then we have a provincial minister of health. We have many deputies. We have the universities, colleges and hospitals training the health care workers. Who is responsible for what and where are the problems? There are loud and frequent complaints that health care is costing too much. Is that a fair complaint? Does health care cost more per capita in Quebec than in Ontario, or more in Canada than in another country? Do we have figures that can be compared? If we don't have the figures, why don't we have them? How do our costs compare with those of other countries? And where, exactly, are our costs out of line? Is it with the doctors, or is it in nursing, or administration, or drugs, or what? Why don't we have figures that can be looked at and discussed?

It is widely recognized that health care for a serious problem is addressed quite well in all of Canada. When there is a need for a cardiac stent or a by-pass operation it is done promptly with no hold-up. If the need is for a knee replacement or a routine colonoscopy, though, the waiting period can be unacceptably long, possibly over a year. Can that be fixed, or need that be fixed?

I believe that efficiency can be built into the system by more appropriate rewards. Institutions and doctors who do more and do it well should be rewarded more than institutions and doctors who do less, have more complications, or attract more complaints. We must bring back recognition for work done well. Why would that be so difficult to do?

There is a problem when patients wait ten hours to be seen at the hospital emergency room. There is a problem if patients wait months for a hip or knee replacement. There is a problem if patients wait months to years to get a replacement family doctor as appears to be the case.

As a rule, patients with an acute problem, like an appendicitis, are taken to the operating room before they perforate and develop serious complications. The problems we have with our health care coverage is distorted by the media. By and large it is not bad. The occasional slip up may and do occur, but the inexcusable delay gets exaggerated publicity because acceptable care is not newsworthy.

But, health care can be improved!

Before I make further suggestions, though, let me mention two books both by academics on the subject. The first, called "Redefining Health Care" was written by Michael E. Porter and Elizabeth Olmstead Teisberg and was published in 2006. It is a 400 page critique of health care in the USA and proposes healthy competition as the solution to its many problems. I am not sure they have it right. The USA is a powerful nation, but its gun laws and overall health care are downright ridiculous. Is it because "the rich and powerful" are unaffected. The second book, called "Managing the Myths of Health Care" is by Henry

Mintzberg, a McGill professor, and was published in 2017.

This is a highly readable 200 page book that examines health care under Medicare in Canada. In a nutshell and in his own words, Mintzberg says the system "reorganizes relentlessly, measures like mad, promotes a heroic form of leadership, favors competition where there is a need for cooperation, and pretends that this CALLING should be managed like a business." Bravo – right on! "Care, cure, control, and community have to collaborate," he says. That is strikingly alliterative, but I prefer health promotion, specific prevention, early diagnosis and treatment, disease limitation, rehabilitation, and palliative care as the logical steps in health care.

I have suggested before how stringent the requirements are to be accepted into medical school, and the standards for the training of our specialists are also exceedingly high and must remain so. But, look at the demographics. It is a fact that doctors are more and more often female to-day than in the past. Fifty years ago, when I was a student, we had about a half a dozen females in a class of just over one hundred. To-day the medical class is about fifty percent female. There is nothing wrong with that: brute strength is not a necessary requirement for medical practice. It is a fact of life, though, that women do not work as many years in practice compared to men. I don't know the reason for that. It may be because of pregnancies, children, family or, perhaps, something else. That is not the point. If more of our doctors are going to be female, and if females have shorter working careers, it means we have to produce more doctors. Who can argue with that?

The doctors' role is also changing. But, many of the things they used to do can be done by nurse practitioners. Why can we not expand that role? Overall, it should bring down the cost of health care and not increase or worsen it. And, computer technology has not yet been fully integrated into medical practice. There may be privacy issues here but, overall, I don't mind if health care workers have access my medical history, the medications I take, the allergies I may have. There can be a category for private information, (like being HIV positive, as an example,) which could be placed under more stringent control. It can also be argued that privacy issues should take a back seat to concerns for the entire population.

If I am caught driving too fast on the high-way, or wobbling too much as I drive, I may be stopped by a police car. I will be asked to show my driver's licence and the car registration. The officer will check the computer and will know in an instant if anything is amiss. Perhaps, in similar fashion, when a patient presents himself to a health care facility he should be asked to show his health card which should be continuously updated with new information, like current medications, results of tests, etc. Inevitably there will be complaints of privacy invasion. That can be debated, but invasion of privacy cuts two ways.

My brother, a retired general surgeon once reprimanded family members for not informing him that the patient who required an emergency appendectomy was HIV positive. He was shocked to learn that the family didn't know that either.

I have a similar tale to tell:

On the morning of the proposed surgery (radical prostatectomy for prostate cancer) my chief resident informs me that the patient, a school teacher, is gay. "I asked him if we could do HIV testing on him but he declined. Will we proceed, nevertheless?" "If you're game, I'm game," I said, or something to that effect. As it turned out, that case happened to be the exceptional one where the resident is splashed in the eyes from washings from the patient's wound, and I get pricked by a needle.

I asked for the patient's blood to be tested for HIV right away.

"I don't care what laws I am breaking: do the test," I said. After the operation, I sent a note to the hospital lawyer.

The hospital policy that allows patients to decline HIV testing is putting me and my surgical team at risk, I said in the note. Should anyone of us be rendered HIV positive because of the hospital policy I will hold you liable.

The hospital lawyer rushed to see me. "You didn't mean this, did you?" the lawyer asked.

"If I didn't mean it, I would not have sent it," I replied.

The hospital policy was changed some time later. I don't know if my note had anything to do with it. As I understand it, the blood test can now be done without the patient's consent and the results not shared with the patient if that is what he wishes. The point is this: if the patient's blood is HIV positive, and if anybody in the health-care team is exposed to that blood directly, as by a hollow needle prick, immediate treatment can abort a transmission. Fortunately for all of us, the patient's blood test came back HIV negative.

Years before this episode I remember one of our resident doctor contracted hepatitis from a patient. That almost killed him. An orthopedic surgeon friend had to suspend practice for some time after a hepatitis transmission during surgery. There was a newspaper account of a lady pediatric surgeon in Montreal whose life was taken by an operating room transmission of a deadly virus. Working in health care has its hazards.

With the technology we have to-day it should be made possible to access information on any citizen with a legitimate health card. The data should be continuously updated so that upon presentation to a health care facility, like a hospital or a doctor's office, the background medical history, current medications, allergies, etc., can be accessed immediately by the treating team. This could save time and assure more accuracy. Can there be privacy issues? Of course, but abuse of privileged information should be grounds for severe sanctions. Overall, I think it can be made to work.

Already we have "wearables" not unlike a wrist-watch that can monitor a person's blood sugar (HIC's), other standard laboratory blood tests, as well as a cardiogram (ECG) for immediate access by a treating physician. It is still too costly for universal use, but that will change. It is too valuable a tool not to make it universally available to all citizens.

So, how do I envision health care to be structured in Canada?

There should be an all-service 500 bed hospital for every 200,000 citizens. (the population number can be debated up or down.) Each hospital must produce audited, accurate figures available for public consumption: the number of patients seen, the numbers admitted to hospital, the number of different conditions treated, the number of different procedures carried out, outcomes, complication rate, patient satisfaction rate, number of deaths, number of patients transferred out, etc. These numbers should be made available for public scrutiny.

Very expensive medical paraphernalia need not be in every hospital. Resources must be shared. Institutions that do more or are getting better results should be rewarded so that there is an incentive for every institution to do better. There may be a reason why one hospital is getting inferior results: maybe it is saddled with the more complicated cases. A careful audit, at a minimum, is paramount. There must be an incentive, nevertheless, to get good results that stand up to stringent scrutiny.

Let free enterprise and healthy competition thrive. Today we have too many watch dogs pursuing wrongful doings and not enough looking out for performances "beyond the call of duty."

I honestly believe our health care system in Canada is second to none in this world. Add a little incentive and it can be made even better. What we don't need are pompous politicians making silly decisions. We need bright people with integrity running the show. Is that possible? I think so.

I am not sure I have this story right but I will relate it, nevertheless. When the universal Medicare programme was introduced into Canada, the country was going to pay for it, largely, by also introducing a national lottery long considered morally questionable in this "Christian" country. But, when the revenue from the lottery were startlingly profitable, the funds were diverted for other use as well. Am I wrong about this? I could be but I suspect I am not. And, if I am right and if the funds had not been diverted – we might have had the best health care in the world. Sad!

Most complaints about health care in Canada today have to do with access to care than to quality of care. To have access to care the questions that must be asked include the following:

1. Do we have enough health care professionals for the task on hand?
2. How do our numbers compare with those of other countries? Do we have as many cardiologists or urologists per capita, for example, compared to other countries? I was surprised to learn that, per capita, Japan had many more urologists than Canada. My Japanese friends were shocked to observe how hard I worked.
3. Do our professionals work as long or as hard as their counterparts in other countries?
4. Are medical procedures done in a timely fashion? Are the exceptions exaggerated by the media? I am unaware of chemotherapy visits or radiotherapy visits cancelled for no good reason. I am aware of the extraordinary costs of certain medical procedures

but I am unaware of countries that have found a way of doing it for less.

We should develop more practice guidelines. We should have them for all the life threatening problems common to our way of life. Let me illustrate my point with respect to one problem I have dealt with repeatedly in my years of practice. The problem being prostate cancer. Consider a set of identical twins.

One twin(A) is obsessive about his health. He visits his urologist once a year, and gets his annual rectal exam and PSA blood test. At age 64, his PSA has jumped from a reading of 3.7 a year ago to 6.2. He has an MRI (magnetic scan) of the prostate which reveals a suspicious area in his right lobe, gets a MRI guided biopsy, which indicates a Gleason 8 cancer in two of twelve cores. His bone scan is negative. He is offered surgery or radiotherapy as treatment options. He chooses surgery and is cured although he has mild incontinence and moderate erectile dysfunction. He lives a full life and dies of a natural cause at age 87.

The other twin(B) doesn't bother with regular visits or blood testing. At age 67, he develops severe low back pain, sees a naturalist, but with persistent and worsening pain, reluctantly consults a urologist. He has a Gleason 8 cancer that has spread to his back bones, as well as to his ribs and skull. He is started on androgen deprivation therapy, an LHRH analogue called Zoladex. Two years later, his situation is worse. More drugs, including chemotherapy, and palliative radiotherapy are tried but the disease advances and claims his life within another year and a half.

Neither twin had extra insurance coverage.

Which twin has cost the country more?

Let's do the arithmetic.

Twin A will make 35 visits from age 50 to age 85. At $200 for the visit and blood test, this will cost $7,000.00. The MRI and biopsy will cost $4,000. The surgery and hospitalization will cost $30,000.00. This will total $41,000.00.

Twin B will be delinquent with visits so we will not count that. The MRI and biopsy will cost $4.000.00. The hormone therapy will cost $48,000.00. Chemotherapy will cost another $10,000.00. Palliative radiotherapy another $10,000.00. Palliative terminal care will cost another $20.000.00 This will total $92,000.00.

What applies to prostate cancer applies to all the other life-threatening cancers. I am certain people with early diagnosis are more likely to be cured and will cost the country significantly less than people who took their chances, had delayed diagnosis and died despite all efforts to save them. We do need more reliable figures, though, to back up this claim.

CHAPTER SEVEN

Conclusions

So, what have I learned?
1. I must reduce my intake of sugar. That has to be the
   most important lesson. Overall, a 30% reduction
   could result in a 30% increase in life-span. There is
   little doubt that the most toxic product we put into
   our bodies to-day is excess sugar. It is what cigarette
   smoking was a generation ago. We have identified the
   villain – it is sugar and the makers of processed food
   and sweetened beverages. The industry is well aware
   of the fact that we consume much too much sugar.
   Still, they cater to our weakness. They tempt us with
   sweetened carbonated drinks, fully aware that the
   sugar content far exceeds what would be prudent.
   It is criminal because the evidence is overwhelming.
   Would an extra tax on sweetened food and beverages
   solve the problem? Not likely! Incentives have always
   worked better than punishment in changing human
   behaviour. How, then, can we further reward the
   already prudent? Maybe, that is unnecessary. If I was
   to make a suggestion it would be this: allow the upper
   limit of sugar to be "this amount" and any additional
   sweet must be as a sugar substitute.
2. I must learn to meditate and by so doing I should
   expect to lengthen my telomeres. The internet is full

of instructions on how to meditate with minimum effort. I have tried some of them, but it has not yet become a daily habit. I can offer no excuse for that. Meditation and Yoga go hand in hand, in my opinion. I owe it to myself to do it on a regular basis every day. I did go to Yoga sessions offered at the club where I played tennis. The leader was superb, the audience largely female and there was hardly anyone there in my age category. A friend sent me an instruction sheet with ten yoga-type stretching exercises that could be done at home. I bought a yoga mat and started the exercises at home. It has not yet become a daily routine, but I hope to make it so. I feel that the yoga stretches can be done while striving to calm and empty the mind. I can even chant a mantra as I do the stretches.

3. I must exercise a half hour every day: perhaps twenty minutes will suffice. The rewards are substantial and real. I should expect to feel better and live longer. I do enjoy tennis and golf despite the fact that I am mediocre to poor in both activities and, unfortunately, neither are daily events, I must and will get involved with a local gym. I might instead use a part of the basement of my residence as my gym.

4. I shall share as well as give away as much as I can as often as I can as I will reap rewards disproportionate to the sacrifices I make.

5. I must look for the good in people and in the world at large as I will come out ahead of those who are looking in exactly the opposite direction. That does not mean I should abandon any form of "disaster" preparedness. I already have the bottled water,

long acting candles, and tinned sardines.

6. I will continue to encourage and believe in discovery as the route to learning.

7. I feel comfortable promoting the six levels of activities which I believe constitute health care: health promotion, specific prevention, early diagnosis and treatment, disease limitation, rehabilitation, and palliative care. All of health care falls under this umbrella, in my estimation. I need to explore more how much we spend as a nation on the different aspects of health care, and how our expenditures compare with other countries.

8. I know I will see more and better immunotherapy and stem-cell treatment in my lifetime. I hope for a break-through in the understanding and management of Alzheimer's disease. It is long overdue. I hope people of means, like those managing the Gates Foundation, will encourage "older folks" to change the world for the better. Youth must be served, but innovative thinking is not necessarily confined to the young. The world is still run by senior citizens, unfortunately, not necessarily wise-old-men.

9. I will continue to keep an open mind about "magical" products. In my estimation the only one worthy of serious consideration at this time is metformin. I have started it. One 500 mg tablet twice a day is what I have decided to take.

10. I continue to treasure my family. My wife, Joan, originally a nurse and a Newfoundlander has stuck with me for 57 years so far. Our four children and six grand-children are blessings I cherish with all my heart.

11. Longevity is a curse if you don't learn how to best enjoy it.

That is my offering to you and to myself. It begins at the beginning and it ends with my very last breath – Namaste.

A Q&A with Dr. Yosh Taguchi

1. **If you had 3 minutes to convey something to someone who has passed from this world, what would you say, who would it be?**

   If I had just three minutes to say something, it would be to thank my parents for deciding to stay in Canada for the sake of the children at the end of World War II. They had a home and farm in Japan and could have lived comfortably there. They thought the future was brighter for their three children in Canada and stayed despite an unfair treatment from the Canadian government.

2. **What does it feel like to save a life and how many lives would you say you have saved?**

   I practiced my craft to the best of my ability and honestly believed that every patient I looked after was better off under my care. That sounds a little boastful but I honestly believed it.

3. **What was one of your greatest teaching moments?**

   I used to give a one hour lecture to second year students on what Urology was all about. I said some outlandish things but I was never reprimanded for it. For example, I would say: where did the Almighty go wrong in designing the human urinary system?

Well, in women, He should have stuck to His original plan, which was to have women urinate through their belly button, and to close off the bladder neck. That design would have lessened their chances of urinary infections or having urinary incontinence, though you may not like peeing out of your belly button. In men, it made no sense whatsoever to wrap the prostate gland around the urethra. If the prostate was a gland with a separate channel to the urinary passage, all blockages would have been eliminated, and a cancer in the gland would have been easy to remove. At the same time, the gradient for urinary concentration is very efficient and ingenious. I used to have fun with the students and many came to talk to me afterwards. Some became urologists.

4. **What memorable encounters have you had with students?**
A number of them came to me after a lecture to thank me for looking after their father or uncle. One student, I recall, introduced himself as the son of my teacher in 1945, in the war camp in BC. Another Introduced himself as the son of a dear friend. He wanted a vasectomy because he didn't want children in this ugly world. I talked him out of it. I'm glad I did!

5. **What was the most common question your patients asked you over the years?**
What made you stay in Québec? I like French-Canadians. They are among the most tolerant people I know.

6. How do you define love?

When you treasure their lives as much as your own. I feel that way about my wife, children and grandchildren.